FrameWork

for the

SHOULDER

A 6-STEP PLAN FOR
PREVENTING INJURY AND ENDING PAIN

NICHOLAS A. DiNUBILE, MD
with Bruce Scali

RODALE.

Notice

This book is intended as a reference volume only, not as a medical manual.
The information given here is designed to help you make informed decisions about your health.
It is not intended as a substitute for any treatment that may have been prescribed by your doctor.
If you suspect that you have a medical problem, we urge you to seek competent medical help.

The information in this book is meant to supplement, not replace, proper exercise training.
All forms of exercise pose some inherent risks. The editors and publisher advise readers to take
full responsibility for their safety and know their limits. Before practicing the exercises in this book,
be sure that your equipment is well maintained, and do not take risks beyond your level of experience,
aptitude, training, and fitness. The exercise and dietary programs in this book are not intended as a substitute
for any exercise routine or dietary regimen that may have been prescribed by your doctor.
As with all exercise and dietary programs, you should get your doctor's approval before beginning.

Mention of specific companies, organizations, or authorities in this book does not imply
endorsement by the author or publisher, nor does mention of specific companies, organizations,
or authorities imply that they endorse this book, its author, or the publisher.

Internet addresses and telephone numbers given in this book were accurate at the time it went to press.

Rodale books may be purchased for business or promotional use or for special sales.
For information, please write to:
Special Markets Department, Rodale Inc., 733 Third Avenue, New York, NY 10017.

Printed in the United States of America

Rodale Inc. makes every effort to use acid-free ⊗, recycled paper ♺.

Illustrations by Michael Gellatly

Photographs by Mitch Mandel

Library of Congress Cataloging-in-Publication Data

DiNubile, Nicholas A.
    Framework for the shoulder : a 6-step plan for preventing injury and ending pain / Nicholas A. DiNubile.
        p.   cm.
    Includes index.
    ISBN 978-1-60529-592-3 paperback
    1. Shoulder—Wounds and injuries—Exercise therapy.   2. Shoulder—Wounds and injuries—Prevention.   I. Title.
RD557.5.D555   2011
617.5'72044—dc23

                                                                                             2011030162

Distributed to the trade by Macmillan
2   4   6   8   10   9   7   5   3   1   paperback

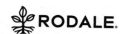

We inspire and enable people to improve their lives and the world around them.
www.rodalebooks.com

To my dream team:

Marybeth, Emily, and Dylan

CONTENTS

PREFACE

Every book in this series has been special to me, and this one is no exception. I've long held the belief that the shoulder is one of the last frontiers of orthopaedic knowledge. We're crossing that frontier now, and I'm thrilled to tell you all about it.

Until recently, the shoulder had been poorly understood. The way my colleagues and I saw things, doctors hadn't come very far from our orthopaedic residency days decades ago, when we had a pretty good knowledge base of common conditions like fractures but didn't fully understand the true functional anatomy of the shoulder or its biomechanics. The arthroscope, the miracle operating tool that enabled us to do delicate, noninvasive repairs, was just being introduced when I was a resident; it exploded onto the scene shortly afterward and was used big-time to advance our knowledge of knees and then elbows, but the shoulder remained a bit of a puzzle.

Three things happened that changed the orthopaedic playing field. First, the arthroscope kept advancing, and the shoulder was the next big joint that it went to. Being able to look closely into every part of it provided firsthand knowledge of how it works, what goes wrong with it, and what's really going on when there's pain. It's a whole lot better than the early years, when all we had to go on was a physical exam and some x-rays.

Second, MRI scanners enabled doctors to see soft tissues, the rotator cuff, the labrum, and other stabilizing structures and begin to understand how they change with age. We can see all sorts of things in the shoulder now that we never fully appreciated before when it comes to both health and injury.

Last, I think we got really good at biomechanical analysis, which is made possible by high-speed video studies being done by trailblazers like Dr. James Andrews and his head therapist, Kevin Wilk.

Thanks to these advances, we now know how the shoulder *works*, and, more important, how and why it *fails*.

A STEPCHILD NO LONGER

The knowledge from recent advances is evolving, and more and more orthopaedic surgeons are opting for a shoulder specialty, adding to the army of shoulder gurus that has sprung up around the land.

No question about it: We're learning more and more about the shoulder, much as we're still learning about the knee. Arthroscopic techniques and tools specifically for the shoulder's structure and components have gotten fairly sophisticated in a very short period of time, and it seems as though every month brings another breakthrough. Patients are getting better results for shoulder complaints because we doctors understand shoulder-disease processes and breakdowns better. We're better at fixing them, better at managing them, and better at *preventing* them.

For me, the shoulder is miles away from where it was not too long ago. It is front and center now, and we're seeing a lot more surgeries—which is okay as long as they are being done by specialists who know how to

JOINT DISCUSSION

I was already well on the road to becoming a knee-centric guy when the shoulder started to become a joint a doctor wanted to be good at. My best friend at that time was Dr. Marty Coleman, a superb orthopaedic surgeon. Marty wanted to apply his finely honed technical skills to the shoulder and talked me into attending a cutting-edge course on shoulder arthroscopy, which at that time was a new, rapidly evolving procedure and discipline.

I had fun with it, working with my good buddy as he enhanced his skills, but down the road, when I started operating on knees only, I sent all my shoulder cases to Marty, who had become a noted shoulder specialist. Unfortunately, Marty moved to greener pastures in Virginia when our Philadelphia area became a pretty terrible environment to work in because of malpractice insurance issues. I still refer shoulder cases because, as I say, I'm a knee-centric guy. If you have a shoulder issue, find yourself a guy like Marty.

navigate around the major arteries and nerves in the shoulder, avoiding major trouble that can occur if an instrument finds its way to the wrong spot. Similar to other specialties in orthopaedics, technology and surgical instrumentation have caught up with the expanded knowledge base, allowing for more and more sophisticated work to be done to repair damaged, unstable, or worn shoulders.

"FRAMING" THE TOPIC

The two previous books in this series were about the lower back and the knee. When I started working on this installment, it struck me that I've had my share of problems with those two areas (for the uninitiated, I'm paying for the athletic exploits of my youth and the resultant traumatic injuries that weren't treated as well as they are today), but I've always had an upper body that could withstand anything, and I never had any real issues with my shoulders. More recently, however, I've realized that I'm a lot closer to the material in this book than I had thought. Having aged a few decades since my quarterbacking days, and because I still have a passion for competitive sports that I pursue on the tennis court, I now see some early warning signs of shoulder issues.

Those issues will have nothing to do with traumatic injury and everything to do with what I have been saying all along: We humans have outlived our frame's warranty. It wasn't designed for a 100-year-old person, let alone one who reaches 120, which is on the horizon for more of us every day.

Like gray hair and wrinkles, age-related changes happen to everyone, and it's almost guaranteed that your shoulders will be markedly different at the age of 40 or 50 from the ones you had when you were 20. What goes on in the upper body is similar to what happens in the lower back and knee: Muscle tissue begins its gradual loss and collagen develops age-related changes, resulting in connective tissue that is less pliable and more brittle and vulnerable. In the shoulder, this affects the rotator cuff (especially its tendons) and the labrum. Also, the neck and cervical spine area undergo degenerative changes that can have a tremendous negative trickle-down impact on shoulder function. Critically, the shoulder and similar joints sometimes just don't have as much cushion (articular cartilage, which is that opaque white stuff on the end of a chicken bone that some of your bones also have, and the labrum, which is soft, spongy tissue akin to a meniscus) as they used to, and arthritis can set in. While shoulder arthritis is not as common as knee or hip arthritis, we are seeing much more of it than ever before.

Everybody is vulnerable to a "pop" in a shoulder as a result of a sudden movement while doing a simple daily task or as a consequence of strenuous recreational activity, and the incidence of shoulder problems is already right up there with knee and lower-back complaints. It is also a fact that shoulders are more problematic for those of us who engage in certain sports and other exercise on a regular basis (especially weight lifting and overhead sports like baseball, tennis, volleyball, and water polo)—but that doesn't mean you shouldn't start exercising your shoulders or should stop working out and playing sports to hedge against your chances of injury.

Quite the contrary, in fact.

An active life is the prescription for extending the frame's warranty, something else I've

JOINT DISCUSSION

Until recently, I could do pretty much anything I wanted without worrying about my shoulders. Back, yes—knees, too, plenty of worries—but not my shoulders. I'd had only one shoulder episode as a young adult, when I may have slightly subluxed (more on that later) one skiing, but it felt fine the next day. I never had a traumatic injury—rotator cuff tear, fractured shoulder, or dislocated shoulder—that debilitates in the long term. The one that did happen to my shoulder was when I shattered my right collarbone in high school fooling around with one of my friends in the neighborhood, but it healed fully without any problems. I sure paid a huge price for that escapade when I missed my entire JV football season at Central High School in Philadelphia. (The silver lining of not getting to throw a single pass or make one tackle that year was that I did help the team as a "trainer," my first foray into sports medicine.)

Now, however, if I do certain things at the gym that I've always done, I have some discomfort, even pain at times. Age and overuse are catching up with me, and I know my rotator cuff is beat up and has started to fray. Going forward, I'll have to be every bit as proactive with my shoulders as I've been with my back and my knees.

been saying all along. The only way you can avoid shoulder problems that come with age, overcome a shoulder complaint faster and with a better outcome, or put off the injuries that come with spirited tennis, golf, and other exercise is to take care of your shoulders *now*. A comprehensive but simple six-step plan for how that should be done is what this book is all about.

TIMELESS ADVICE

Medical knowledge and skills advance all the time, but some recommendations are never out of vogue. My first book, *FrameWork,* presented a global plan for healthy muscles, bones, and joints and introduced a philosophy that will stand for as long as we are built the way we are: To have a long—and active—life, you must exercise every part of your body's structure, and you must *balance* each individual area with the whole (your frame) that it is connected to.

You also need to do it differently at different age points in your life—this is increasingly important as the average age of gymgoers keeps rising. These individuals are bringing their "weak links" to the gym, and many are getting into trouble with their workouts. Fortunately, age-specific training is something personal trainers and fitness professionals have begun to understand. The American Council on Exercise (ACE) recognizes age dynamics and has developed advanced certification programs for its fitness professionals based upon my Frame-Work philosophy and books. This will enable trainers and therapists to design appropriate fitness programs for adults and to modify those programs for the most common orthopaedic ailments.

Part of what we doctors have learned about the shoulder is that it's more susceptible to imbalances in strength and flexibility than any other joint. As a result of treating injuries that afflict top athletic competitors, we know that violent repetitive motions, like pitching a baseball or serving a tennis ball, build up muscle in one area at the expense of another. Sooner or later, unequal forces end up breaking something.

Of import to everyone, however, is that serious athletes aren't alone when it comes to having imbalances. A lot of exercise routines that people swear by, including some "functioning training" programs that are so popular today, and the recreation they pursue end up creating the unequal stresses and imbalances that should be avoided. Too many regular folks who have a laudable dedication to fitness build "mirror muscles" in the gym, or run or bicycle for days and miles on end, without alternating workouts to shore up weaker areas and address the imbalances that their favorite activity or workout has created. Too many of us beat ourselves up on a regular basis, and we too often complicate the imbalance issue by not including proper warmup and recovery.

Proper exercise (and the good health and long life that come with it) starts from the ground up and works the legs, core, and upper body. It starts with foot position, the way a boxer starts a punch with his feet. He doesn't just rely on his shoulder and wing it; he

JOINT DISCUSSION

I'm a USPTA (United States Professional Tennis Association) member and have taken the necessary steps to be a recreational coach. (I'm not a certified pro because I had another calling.) I treat a lot of tennis players, and I have a real soft spot for tennis pros who call my office. I see them primarily for knee issues, but if they want to come in for elbows or other things, I'm happy to examine them and point them in the right direction.

Professional and high-level tennis players will sometimes suffer an acute injury, such as a severe ankle sprain, but their orthopaedic complaints invariably stem from the constant pounding their frame parts take. The game has gotten so much faster and harder; the serves these people hit put maximum torque and other stresses on body parts that weren't exactly designed for them. John McEnroe, a Hall of Fame champion who is still a competitive player on the Masters circuit and in World Team Tennis (and an awesome tennis commentator to boot), has said he would love to have the serve that some of the current *women* players have.

The way tennis is played today—a power game with much higher forces as a result of new strings and rackets—it's not just tennis elbow anymore. We're seeing a lot more significant wrist and shoulder injuries that cause pros to lose playing time. Juan Martín del Potro, after winning the US Open in 2009, was out for more than 9 months with a wrist injury that required surgery, and given the practice and rigorous tournament sched-

marshals the power of his legs and his trunk to deliver a mighty blow. He relies on the biomechanical link from foot to fist.

We doctors rely on that video analysis mentioned above to establish baselines of peak performance. We use that knowledge to design the best exercise program, and we combine it with other diagnostics to identify a breakdown and the best treatment for it. Whether your goal is to be in the best possible shape or to come back from a shoulder injury, you simply must work your entire frame, and keep working it. If you don't stay on top of every frame part, something will surely get out of whack later.

Or sooner.

ules pros play, it's a wonder many more of them aren't on the shelf. We are also seeing more and more hip problems, knee tendinitis, and leg stress fractures than we ever have. Rafael Nadal, with his pounding, aggressive, all-out, never-give-up style of play, is beginning to break down more frequently, even at his young age.

I like to think that the best nutrition and training regimens could solve this, but I wonder at times if some of the newer training routines are not part of the problem. The "What doesn't kill you makes you stronger" attitude may also be in play when it comes to many orthopaedic problems in competitive sports and high-level athletes. The cycle of fitness training, sport-specific practice, and competition results in cumulative stresses that can expose one's "weak links" that result in breakdown.

It's vital to know that musculoskeletal stresses accumulate silently, and overload can sneak up on you. Even recreational players aren't immune to repetitive-use injuries, tennis elbow and the like, that have been around forever. Had I the time, I could fill an entire schedule with just shoulder or elbow complaints that take those patients out of their game. Whatever your game is, you will have a better chance of avoiding debilitating injury if you get on the best nutrition and training regimen at your disposal.

Train hard, fuel yourself, and allow adequate rest and recovery. This is the recipe for true gains, without loss.

JOINT DISCUSSION

Swimmers are notoriously overtrained, and their practice routines create predictable imbalances. They're in the water so much, and yet, as a rule, swim coaches think their charges need to swim more. (To be fair, wrestling coaches think their grapplers should wrestle more, track coaches think their teams need to run more—coaches of other sports pretty much recommend more of whatever they teach.) Ironically, it's not unusual to hear stories about swimmers who missed training for a week because of the flu or a cold and then set world-record times shortly after getting back into the water. They had the skills and conditioning; they just needed a little recovery time to show their full potential.

There's just too much training and not enough recovery and cross-training going on at every level of sports and physical exercise. Johnny Weissmuller, the world-famous swimmer who won five gold medals and 52 US national championships, setting 67 world records along the way, said he never had a problem with his rotator cuff until he started swinging from trees as Tarzan on the big screen. That puzzled him, because he thought he had been moving his upper body much as he had in the pool.

I have no idea if Johnny knew how lucky he was not to have shoulder problems as a swimmer, but I can assure you that he, along with his trainers and doctors, had no clue about the critical factors that contributed to the shoulder condition he had as an actor. How could they? We didn't know until long after he died in 1984 that frame parts are different for everyone—from couch potato to world-class athlete—well before middle age. Years of swimming and overuse were his "setup," and his weak link was exposed by the combination of swinging in the trees and Father Time's aging process.

Johnny's shoulders were different when he retired from swimming.

Your shoulders will be different in the days to come.

Engage the changes going on in your frame, or cast your lot with Lady Luck.

SHOULDER THIS

I've consulted with and treated many celebrities and sports stars. But those who have read my previous books know that I only mention people like Arnold Schwarzenegger because what they've experienced medically has great value to everybody. In that vein, there's a particular world-class sports-medicine encounter in my past that has a real connection to this book's subject.

In June of 2004, I was in Texas to speak at a medical conference. During breaks I always try to work out in the hotel gym, and while riding a stationary bike during one particular session on that trip, I spied some tennis magazines in a wall rack.

It was right before Wimbledon, and I had just gotten back into serious tennis after a 15-year hiatus when, for all intents and purposes, I had been out of the tennis loop. The cover story of a magazine that caught my eye was about an almost totally unknown 17-year-old female player who had a Russian name and played a two-handed game. She was stunning, too, I might add, but that wasn't the reason I almost fell off my stationary bike. *Could she be the child prodigy I'd consulted with 7 years ago?*

I thumbed the magazine in a hurry and scanned the article, and the coincidences mounted up. The young woman was represented by IMG and trained at the famous Nick Bollettieri Tennis Academy, two of the "players" involved in the case from my past. What stuck out most of all was that she was a right-handed player who, as the article pointed out, was so ambidextrous that when she first came to the USA, there was serious consideration of making her a lefty, as lefties have clear advantages in the sport.

My mind flashed back 7 or 8 years to a call I received from a sports agent at IMG about an 8- or 9-year-old tennis phenom and her father, who had been told by a touring world-famous female tennis champion 5 years previously that his 5-year-old daughter was extraordinary and that he should do "everything he could to get this kid to the US for lessons and coaching."

As the story goes, it took Dad those 5 years to scrape together the money for two airfares (Mom had to be left behind) to the States. As soon as they landed, they headed—unannounced—straight to the Bollettieri Academy office, where Dad pleaded for someone to evaluate and train his daughter. Apparently Bollettieri saw enough to take them under his wing.

So there I was, consulting with those responsible for a very young Russian female player who had phenomenal skills and the makings of a champion. Her advisors told me that the girl had played as a righty ever since she'd started hitting tennis balls at around age 4, but they suspected she was a natural lefty. (They also mentioned in passing Dad's recurring dream of seeing his daughter winning a major championship playing left-handed.) Apparently the advisors had seen an interview with me in the *Wall Street Journal* about eye dominance in sports. They wanted to find out for sure about the girl's natural hand dominance, and whether they should consider having her switch hands.

I also learned that Dad and daughter were living in a motel, he was driving a taxi and was barely able to make ends meet, and resources for medical evaluation were lim-ited. I told them that the facility I had at the time was a certified Olympic testing site with every piece of equipment imaginable, and yes, some tests could be done. I assured them that I'd do everything within my power to get as much as possible free of charge for Dad and his little girl.

They were posing two very interesting questions: whether one could know what one's natural dominance side is, and whether one could know if it had been switched at a young age. Depending on the outcome of tests, the question was whether she could be switched back without upsetting the apple cart.

Before starting any evaluations, however, I wanted to be honest about what doctors, athletic trainers, and exercise physiologists knew and didn't know about the subject. I told them about my own experience with ambidextrous-

JOINT DISCUSSION

The question of hand dominance is an interesting one, especially for me. I was one of those lefties who had been converted as a kid; whenever I picked up something with my left hand, my parents and the nuns at Catholic school would always put it in the other one. I can't say that being "righted" was a pleasant experience, but it turned out to be a blessing in disguise, because I am fairly ambidextrous and much more effective as a surgeon in the operating room.

ness, which had spurred a keen interest in hand dominance. (In fact, I had wanted to go beyond hand dominance to find out if leg and arm dominance coincide with the hand. I was certain biomechanical aficionados in the sports world—and other doctors—would want to know that, too.) I informed my inquirers that I had called around to some of the smartest people I knew, but none of them could tell me there was conclusive testing for hand dominance, let alone leg or arm. Regardless, I told them I'd be delighted to run some sophisticated tests on her and try to figure out what her natural side was.

And then I had to be right up-front about something else: I already knew what my recommendation was going to be.

Leave her alone.

I told them that although I hadn't been able to get a consensus from the experts, I had come to one conclusion after years of orthopaedic practice: People get wired early in terms of neuromuscular learning, especially as it applies to sports. Their young client had been playing the same way since she was 4 or 5. If she's looking that good, I told them, don't disrupt it. (Her situation was different from that of Rafael Nadal, a natural righty playing left-handed. As a youngster, he hit two-handed forehand and backhand until he was around 9 years old, as it became common for children to learn tennis initially hitting two-handed from both sides. His very wise uncle and coach Toni, well aware of the lefty advantage, had Rafa start hitting his powerful forehands left-handed as he and his game matured.)

The girl's advisors thanked me, said they'd let Dad know how I felt, and get back to me.

I never heard back from them.

I hadn't thought about them until I picked up that tennis magazine in the hotel gym many years later. I couldn't resist the urge to find out whether that unknown young star was the little girl I had possibly influenced long before, so I made an inquiry when I got home.

The nice folks at IMG informed me that the girl and her agent had just left for Wimbledon, but that they'd follow up with me upon return.

There was no way I'd miss watching Wimbledon that year. I observed as best I could the 17-year-old girl hitting as a right-hander with an awesome two-handed backhand. On occasion, when she was out of position and was forced to react in a hurry, she'd hit a left-handed forehand, but it was obvious to me that she was a natural righty. I remember thinking, if this was the same girl, I'd made the right decision in her case. If she was the same girl whose father had pulled out all the stops to get her there, I also knew where her tremendous heart and fight came from. Like millions of fans around the world, I was thrilled when I saw her capture the Wimbledon title. I've been a big fan ever since.

I don't think I would have gotten a call back from the girl's IMG agent if I hadn't called days before the whole world was introduced to Maria Sharapova. They probably would have thought I was some kook who had seen her on TV. But I had made the call before she starred in Wimbledon, so the agent called me back. After I recapped my story, he said it could very well be true that she and the girl I'd advised were one and the same. He said he wasn't her agent back then and would get back to me after he looked into it.

Sure enough, my suspicion proved correct. I thought that would be the end of the story.

Flash forward a few years, which was a couple of years ago. Maria was in the Philadelphia area, playing a tournament at Villanova, minutes from my home, and there was no way I'd miss it. As she had been having some minor knee problems, this knee guy also wanted to weigh in, so I placed another call to her agent. He was very gracious to return it, and we exchanged a few calls, hoping to all get together after the match.

It didn't work out. Doctor that I am, I couldn't conclude our final conversation without mentioning some imbalances around her shoulder I'd noticed while attending the Villanova match. (That's one of the problems with being a sports doc with an interest in biomechanics. It's hard for me to watch an athlete or dancer without spotting potential issues.) I was worried that they could be a source of problems in the future. The agent thanked me for my unsolicited advice, and we hoped to touch base again in the future.

Which brings us to the value of this particular encounter.

A few years after that conversation, Sharapova started having some really serious shoulder problems, to the point that her career was threatened. She ended up having shoulder surgery and had to do some intensive rehabbing afterward.

I'm not a psychic, I'm a doctor. I can't stop helping someone if I'm in a position to help, which is why I picked up the phone again and contacted the IMG agent when Maria was still in rehab. I told him that I knew she was in good hands for her orthopaedic care and rehabilitation, but I couldn't help pointing out shoulder-height differences and the forward posture of her dominant shoulder, indicating both tightness and weakness in the rotator cuff and rhomboids (muscles near the scapula, or "wing bone") that I had noticed in her over the years. I also wondered aloud if some of her fitness and training routines were contributing to the imbalances and overload that she was experiencing. I added that it might be efficacious to include the FrameWork approach to her recovery program. Whatever she was doing, I told him, it should deal with the imbalances created by playing tennis day in and day out, the same way that baseball pitchers have to work really hard on their throwing-side shoulders—front-to-back, side-to-side, and up-down. Again he thanked me for my concern and input and assured me that she was on the road to recovery.

What should you take from this story?

Your body adapts to the physical stresses you place on it. Not all of the adaptations are necessarily good ones. Constantly checking for imbalances in your frame is essential. Your body will also sometimes begin to cheat in terms of movement patterns, masking imbalances until breakdown occurs. Injuries don't always come out of the blue; some are *very* predictable. And that brings us to one of my favorite medical recommendations, one that is always in vogue but not practiced enough, even by the medical community: An ounce of prevention is worth a pound of cure.

PLAN TO BE HEALTHY

It doesn't matter who you are, or at what level you recreate, exercise, or play sports. If every part of your frame isn't in shape and balanced with the other parts it's connected to, you're asking for trouble. The good news is that it really isn't all that hard to accomplish, and all it takes is six steps.

Step 1 is learning about the major components of your shoulder and its support staff (upper back, cervical spine, core, et al.) and how they work and contribute to motion, function, and performance. Exercises are always more tolerable—and easier to stick with—if you know *why* you're doing them.

Step 2 brings you up to speed on what can go wrong with your shoulders, and what you can do about it.

Step 3 is a short shoulder-related self-test that shines some light on your overall health, your weak links, and what kind of shape your frame is in.

Step 4 is about timeless recommendations for lifestyle and general fitness issues. This is the foundation for extending your frame's warranty.

Step 5 is where the rubber meets the road. You'll work your shoulders as never before to combat age-related changes going on there, to prevent serious injury down the road, and to recover faster and better should an injury show up.

Step 6 is full of prescriptions for problematic shoulders. No matter what, there's always something you can do to make things better. Forewarned is forearmed, and that's pretty critical when it comes to your health. If you're for-tunate not to need extra help right now, count your blessings and pass on any nuggets that might just help a buddy who has a bum wing.

There you have it. All you need to get *going*. A short **Afterword** puts a bow on things with some tidbits about what the future will look like when it comes to shoulders. It's a window onto the imminent crossing of one of those final frontiers of orthopaedics. With the trusty arthroscope in hand, and procedures such as shoulder replacements one day becoming as commonplace as those for the knee and hip, it's sooner than you think.

Shoulder on: It's again time to get *active for life*.

SHOULDER THIS

As with the other books in the FrameWork series, the "frame" part of the program comes before the "work" part. The first step toward healthy shoulders is learning about the form and function—the biomechanics—that are responsible for the *action* in an active life.

Although I'm primarily a "knee guy," the shoulder intrigues me to no end and I keep my finger, if not my scalpel and arthroscope, on a truly unique joint whose balance of mobility versus stability is unmatched anywhere else in the body. Although there is some rotation in the knee, it's more like a hinge: It places a premium on front-to-back movement, and stability is more important than additional rotational capability. Its ligaments lock things down pretty tight, and the patellofemoral joint is designed primarily to go up and down. The hip is a ball and socket, as the shoulder joint is, but it has a much deeper socket that, again, trades off some mobility for stability. Don't get me wrong—stability is really important in the shoulder—

but you have to give up some stability for the enhanced mobility—*action*—that only the shoulder provides. It goes up and down, side to side, and almost all around.

Perhaps it was an evolutionary thing when we started to come out of the trees; whatever the explanation, what we've got is a humeral head (the ball at the top of the upper arm bone) that sits in the glenoid (a shallow socket at the end of the scapula, or shoulder blade), and the labrum (firm rubbery material akin to menisci in the knee) and articular cartilage (the cushion covering the joint surface) on the ends of bones that prevent bone-on-bone contact through a wide range of motion.

The glenoid is so shallow that only one-third of the humeral head sits in it, so the shoulder is inherently a very mobile joint that, once more, lacks stability. If it's loose, its movement can be like an ice cube on a plate. That's where the capsule—a tricky anatomical construct if ever there was one—and shoulder muscles, tendons, and labrum come into play big-time to keep things in check.

What it all comes down to is that the shoulder relies more on the soft tissue around it than other major joints do. The good news is that muscles are the one part of shoulder anatomy that you can do something about *right now*. The brief primer on anatomical basics that follows will get you started.

THE BARE BONES

Large joints have large bones as a foundation, and the three in your shoulder play a large role in the variable motion it provides:

Clavicle (collarbone): This gently curved bone serves primarily as a strut to which shoulder muscles attach from the sternum (breastbone) and chest area. It is prone to fracture because it is just under the skin.

Scapula (shoulder blade): A thin, flat bone with several prominences (ridges and extensions). I've heard it referred to as the "conductor" of the shoulder because of its

SHOULDER AND CHEST
FRONT VIEW

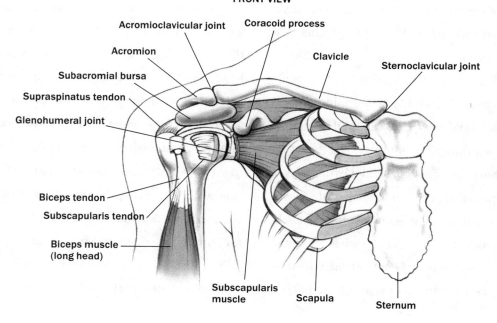

Acromioclavicular joint

Coracoid process

Acromion

Clavicle

Subacromial bursa

Sternoclavicular joint

Supraspinatus tendon

Glenohumeral joint

Biceps tendon

Subscapularis tendon

Biceps muscle
(long head)

Subscapularis
muscle

Scapula

Sternum

importance in shoulder function. Three prominences merit special mention because they are closest to shoulder action: the *acromion* ("peak of the shoulder" in Greek), which narrowly extends from the scapula and then fans out to meet the clavicle at the acromioclavicular, or AC, joint; the aforementioned *glenoid* (shallow cup), just below the acromion; and the *coracoid process*, a sort of hook that helps stabilize things.

Humerus (upper arm bone): Of primary importance in shoulder biomechanics is the humeral head, which has an articular cartilage surface (discussed below) to minimize friction, plus attachment sites for the four rotator cuff tendons (also discussed below). It also helps power the main muscles of the upper arm, including the deltoid, biceps, and triceps.

JOINT CONCERNS

Allow me to say yet again that motion is what FrameWork is all about. If the bones above touched, there wouldn't be much shoulder movement, and what little there was would likely come with quite a bit of pain.

Not touching is one thing; proper separation another. When any space between bones starts to differ from what Mother Nature gave you, beware. You may not have any pain or visible symptoms right away, but initial breakdowns pretty much always get worse, and you'll know about it soon enough.

There are three locations in the shoulder where space between bones is critical:

Glenohumeral Joint: If you envision a golf ball on an oversize tee, you'll get a good idea of what this joint looks like and why the humeral head (the "ball") and the glenoid (the "tee") are stable but free to move in any direction.

Acromioclavicular (AC) Joint: Where the clavicle meets the acromion. Small and hardly mobile, this joint is subject to injury ("AC separation") and arthritis.

Sternoclavicular (SC) Joint: Connects the clavicle to the sternum (middle of the chest).

THE SOFTER SIDE

Now that we've gone through the "hard" stuff, let's explore some other frame parts in your shoulders that have their counterparts in the knee and are just as critical for healthy joint function:

Articular Cartilage

Our old friend that we visited in the knee book—the opaque white stuff that we see on the ends of chicken bones—is back, this time as the head of the humerus and the crater rim of the glenoid. Articular cartilage is smooth material that absorbs shock, and it's slippery, so it keeps friction between touching, moving parts to an absolute minimum. In other words, it allows for smooth and pain-free *articulation*, or motion. It is pretty remarkable stuff; when healthy, it has a coefficient of friction 10 times greater than ice on ice! That's a pretty smooth ride.

Labrum

Akin to the meniscus, this wedge-shaped fibrocartilage ring sits atop the glenoid articular cartilage. The labrum helps to anchor the biceps tendon, cushions the humeral head, and deepens the joint socket, which adds static, or relatively stationary, stability to the shoulder.

Capsule

This frame part, which also provides static stability, is a watertight sac between the glenoid and the humerus that is designed to prevent shoulder instability, such as subluxation and dislocation.

Ligaments

These fibrous bands connect bone to bone:

- **Glenohumeral Ligaments:** They limit excessive sliding and rotation of the humeral head on the glenoid during arm movement—the last leg of the triad that provides static stability to the shoulder.

- **Coracoclavicular Ligaments:** The acromion (the scapula peak) is held in correct relation to the clavicle primarily by these ligaments.

- **Coracoacromial Ligament:** Connects the acromion to the coracoid process (the scapula's "hook"), forming a vault that protects the humeral head, and plays a supporting role to the coracoclavicular ligaments.

- **Acromioclavicular Ligament:** Connects the acromion to the clavicle.

Tendons

These softer tissues are much like ligaments, but they connect bone to muscle instead of bone to bone:

- **Biceps Tendon:** Connects the biceps muscle to the top of the glenoid, and also melds with the labrum.

- **Rotator Cuff Tendons:** Each of the four muscles that make up the rotator cuff (discussed below) has a corresponding tendon that attaches its deepest layers to the humeral head.

Muscles

Muscles provide dynamic, or mobile, stability in the shoulder. Muscle strength has been a cornerstone of the FrameWork philosophy and programs from the start, but muscle balance, especially around the shoulder girdle, is just as important. This is perhaps why shoulder problems rank number one in weight lifters and gym rats, especially men. In their effort to achieve maximum strength and muscular growth, they all too often overwork certain shoulder muscles, do not allow for adequate recovery between workouts, and in the process create fatigue and imbalances, especially in the smaller muscle groups. Muscles are designed to *move*. These are the ones that get your shoulder going, and the ones that will *all* need your attention:

- **Trapezius:** A large, superficial muscle that extends from the occipital bone (back of the head) down to the midback vertebrae and over to the scapula spine (protruding ridge of the backbone). Its primary function is to retract the scapula.

- **Rhomboids:** Smaller muscles in the upper back that originate on the spinal column and attach to the midregion of the scapula. They also function as scapula retractors and are extremely important not only for posture but for optimal shoulder health and function.

- **Serratus Anterior:** Originates on the upper eight or nine ribs at the side of the chest and attaches to the long edge of the scapula below the glenoid.

- **Deltoid:** Powers glenohumeral joint abduction, flexion, and extension. It takes over lifting the arm once it's away from the side.

- **Pectoralis Major:** A thick, fan-shaped muscle that covers much of the upper chest. Its broad side originates in the upper part of the sternum and extends to attach to the clavicle; its tapering side terminates in the upper humerus. The pectorals are powerful abductors and internal rotators of the glenohumeral joint. In layman's terms, they move the arms across the body. Bodybuilders often work their "pecs" with the bench press.

- **Latissimus Dorsi:** The widest and most powerful back muscle. It originates on the lower half of the back at the iliac crest (hip bone) and then tapers to attach to the front of the upper part of the humerus. It also provides abduction and internal rotation, moving the arm downward and backward.

■ **Rotator Cuff:** Last, but certainly not least, is this somewhat infamous frame part that helps to raise the arm from the side and rotates the shoulder in myriad directions. As important as those biomechanical functions are, however, the cuff's primary purpose is to stabilize the humeral head against the glenoid. Unlike the deltoid, it's a very tiny group of four strap muscles that can easily become overworked, imbalanced, and fatigued. (The reason it tears, especially after long-term high-spirited sports and recreation, is that we demand performance that

exceeds design specifications. We'll have plenty to say about this affliction in the next step.) While the deltoid is the *power* mover, the cuff provides *fine-tuned* movement.

The four muscles that make up the cuff and work in concert to activate and protect are:

● **Supraspinatus:** Lies above the scapula spine and attaches along with the infraspinatus muscle on the outer tuberosity (protuberance) of the humeral head. It is active in any motion involving elevation of the humerus, working to stabilize the glenohumeral joint. The supraspinatus is the cuff muscle that tends to get into the most trouble.

● **Infraspinatus:** Also stabilizes the humeral head, and it accounts for 60 per-

MUSCLES OF THE ROTATOR CUFF

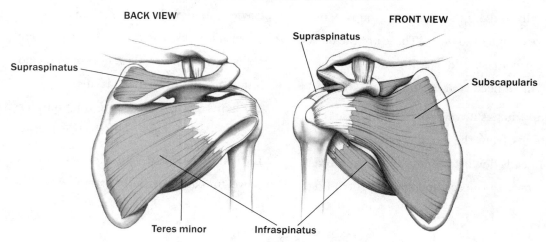

BACK VIEW   FRONT VIEW

Supraspinatus   Supraspinatus

Supraspinatus   Subscapularis

Teres minor   Infraspinatus

cent of external rotation strength at the shoulder.

- **Teres Minor:** Just below the infraspinatus, it provides the remaining 40 percent of external rotation strength at the shoulder.

- **Subscapularis:** The only muscle attaching to the lesser tuberosity of the humeral head; serves as an internal rotator.

Nerves, Blood Vessels, and Bursae

With one exception, all of the important nerves that power the shoulder and transmit messages back to the brain are branches of the brachial plexus, which begins in the spine and also controls elbow, wrist, and hand function. That exception, the cranial nerve that is also known as the spinal accessory nerve, is connected to the trapezius muscle. Blunt force trauma and/or swelling in the shoulder can lead to tingling, numbness, or paralysis—usually temporary—in the shoulder, elbow, or hand. Compression of the suprascapular nerve may result in a motor palsy (also known as muscle weakness) that can mimic a rotator cuff tear. The long thoracic innervates the serratus anterior muscle, which can be prone to stretch injury.

The shoulder is often the source of "referred pain" when nerves are malfunctioning, stretched, or irritated. This is especially true when there is a pinched nerve in the neck: Many patients call the office complaining that they have a shoulder problem or injury. This is why a proper shoulder evaluation always includes the neck or cervical spine area as well as a check of the other nerves mentioned above.

Traveling along with the nerves are the large vessels that supply the arm with blood. Six branches extend from the axillary artery, all of which provide rich collateral circulation to much of the shoulder. (If you place your hand in your armpit, you may be able to feel the pulsing of this large vessel.) Unfortunately, as we learned about the articular cartilage in the knee, the humeral head does not have extensive collateral circulation, and this complicates how fast and how well its injuries heal.

Sandwiched between the rotator cuff muscles and the outer layer of large, bulky shoulder muscles are sacs with small amounts of lubricating fluid that are known as bursae. They are everywhere in the body, including the knee, as we learned, and you'll find them wherever two body parts move against one another and there is no joint to reduce the friction. The shoulder joint, like all synovial joints, also contains a lubricating, nourishing fluid called synovial fluid.

WEAK LINKS

Every health-management or improvement program, especially an exercise one that places additional stresses on the frame, should consider one's predisposition to breakdown. If your family has a history of cardiovascular disease, it's prudent to get on a diet and supplement regimen at an early age to keep cholesterol in check. If breast cancer is the issue, closer monitoring of that tissue is called for. When it comes to working out, one must consider those "setups" for the breakdowns I'm always talking about, which everyone has in one way or another, to one degree or another.

Weak links are one of the common threads in this series because they play a role in every aspect of frame health. Many of them can be corrected by you yourself, and those that are beyond your control can usually be well managed.

Age

First up is something that no one can control forever: the wear and tear on body parts and the changes in tissue composition as time marches on. Friction takes its toll and collagen loses elasticity, so most adults over the age of 40 have rotator cuffs that have already started fraying. We have learned much of this from MRI technology that shows the internal architecture of the cuff and associated tendons—sometimes more than we want to see. Few adults have significant discomfort at first, but the fraying goes on and degenerative scar-type tissue forms within the cuff. Compromised strength and mobility in your shoulder may be slight, even imperceptible at first, but the process can be relentless and unstoppable. (It *can* be minimized, however, hence this program.)

Bones shrink and weaken with age, and women are more prone to deficits than men. Everyone is at higher risk for fractures later in life, and recovering from them is more problematic with each advancing decade. Fractures around the shoulder, especially the upper humerus, are extremely common and can be devastating in terms of functional loss in the shoulder and arm. Osteoporosis (significant bone loss) and osteopenia (early-stage bone loss) are the relentless enemy, but they can be fought. Bone mass is easy to check, and exercise is a proven bone builder, especially when combined with adequate calcium and vitamin D intake (covered in Step 4), so you can be proactive when it comes to your bone health. Ideally, this should start in the teen years, especially for girls. The stronger your bones are going into adulthood, the better off you will fare in mid- and later life in terms of bone health.

Blood vessels also change markedly with age. Although most of the shoulder is well supplied with blood, there are some areas of the rotator cuff, along with the humeral head we mentioned above, that have fewer tributaries. This fact on its own is a concern when it comes to the oxygen and nutrients required for proper function and injury healing; when the potential supply is reduced as a result of vascular decline, injury recovery can be harder, longer, and less than optimum. This is one of the reasons why motion is lotion to the shoulder: Exercise gets blood flowing in the nooks and crannies, the microcirculation networks in muscles and tendons.

All of the above adds up to higher vulnerability. Yessiree—age is a biggie when it comes to weak links, and it's a big part of the next chapter on what can go wrong with our shoulders.

SHOULDER THIS

Consequences of aging that threaten every frame:

■ Probability of injury increases.

■ Severity of injury increases.

■ Time to heal increases.

■ Degree of healing decreases.

■ Cellular and biochemical changes occur:

● Bone loses density.

● Ligaments weaken.

● Growth hormone production decreases.

● Collagen is lost and its structural integrity diminishes.

● Muscle mass and strength diminish, as does reaction time.

● Neural loss (Neuromuscular wiring goes from high-speed cable to dial-up.)

● Loss of proprioception (fine-tuned motion we discussed at length in *FrameWork for the Knee*)

General Health

We know that people with diabetes are more prone to frozen shoulders and rotator cuff issues than the average person, and that being overweight also plays a major role in rotator cuff tears. More recent research on

SHOULDER THIS

tendinopathy (tendon disease) has shown a significant link between high cholesterol and tendon injury, something that had been suspected for some time in Achilles tendinitis cases. A word to the wise: If you're not managing a general health condition well, you're well on your way to a shoulder breakdown.

Lifestyle

First and foremost—because you can do a lot about it—is how much you *move*. Even if you're new to FrameWork, you know that being sedentary is not an option if you want to enjoy the best of health. If you don't do anaerobic exercise on a regular basis, your muscles and bones lose strength at a much higher rate. Skip out on the aerobics and you'll reduce soft-tissue tone, efficiency, and ability to heal, not to mention cardiovascular health.

You can take a hard look at how you sleep, too. If you lie on your side all night, the rota-

JOINT DISCUSSION

I always ask my shoulder patients if they are doing something on a regular basis besides exercise that might explain their discomfort or pain. Anything that requires raising one's elbow above shoulder level and/or craning one's neck (painting a ceiling, trimming a tree, and the like) could be the culprit because the rotator cuff gets pinched repetitively. Whatever you do for recreation or work that involves your shoulders, do it *right*. Ditto for neck use—avoid reading or watching TV for hours in bed with your neck propped at an unnatural right angle. Get lessons from a competent trainer so you can play the right way, and use ladders and other tools to work the right way. Also think about posture and neck position in bed and at the computer, laptop, or tablet (more on this subject later on). If you do, you are much less likely to show up in a doctor's office with a complaint that mystifies you, as many of my patients do.

tor cuff will get irritated, or you can get a kink or pinched nerve in your neck. You might even be cutting off circulation a little bit (and that problem can be exacerbated on a night you drink too much alcohol before bedtime and wind up passed out in one position). This is why a lot of people can't point to why a shoulder hurts and say that they "just woke up that way."

Technological advances that we use every day improve our quality of life immeasurably, but they're not without their pitfalls. Stiff knees, backs, and hips accompany those who sit at desks all day, and barking forearms and wrists pop up with greater frequency everywhere as a result of texting and tweeting and keyboard tapping. There may be no turning back from the miniaturization and speed of communication we now have, but we sure can cut back a tad, take more breaks (find that rest stop off the information highway!), and pay more attention to shoulder, arm, and wrist exercises that provide lotion for those motions.

Joint Laxity

As you've learned, the shoulder is inherently mobile and some people's joints are inherently hypermobile ("looser"). They'll pop when oth-ers' wouldn't during normal basketball or football play or even, in some cases, when doing nothing more than throwing a ball or even returning a glass to a high cabinet. Regardless of when it happens and under what circumstances, it's called a subluxation, and once it pops out a little bit, it stretches farther. It doesn't take too many pops for a full dislocation to become a reality.

Active, but How?

Proper form and technique are always critical when you exercise and play sports, and never more than when it comes to activities that rely heavily on the shoulder. Serving a tennis ball, pitching a baseball, swimming, gymnastics, and volleyball are all examples of how the shoulder is pushed to its design limitations—and beyond, in some cases. Even when perfect form and technique are on display, shoulder problems often arise from the repetitive stress inherent in some sports and recreational activities. Don't let your form and technique become weak links that escalate the risk of debilitation or injury.

And don't let imbalance be a culprit, either. Fitness fanatics who run or work out religiously in the gym, or who hit the courts and playing fields every week, are prone to having an overworked frame part that taxes other ones abnormally. Imbalances develop as a direct result of their activity or sport, something I see all the time. (These imbalances could also result from rehabbing or compensating for an injured part, as in my own case.) Optimal biomechanics relies on form, function, and force; imbalance in any part of the motion equation could break the chain of health at any time. Another word to the wise: Get trained by a competent professional, and get regular tune-ups with him or her.

Old Injuries

Your body is just like paper, metal, and wood: Its cracks, tears, and breaks can be "glued," "taped," "stapled," or "welded," but it may never be as strong as it was originally. If you want to avoid a *Groundhog Day* injury experience, pay special attention to the elements that have an impact on your future mobility:

- Incomplete rehabilitation
- Strenuous recreation: ramped up too soon
- Improper warmup of affected area
- Poor nutritional support
- Overtraining and/or overuse syndromes
- Medication camouflage

SHOULDER THIS

Weak Links

- Aging EFX
- Subpar general health
- Lifestyle
- Joint laxity
- Imbalances (shoulder *and* workouts)
- Old injuries
- Incomplete rehab
- Genetics

All of the above can cut short your recovery, establishing a new baseline that is less than it could have been and that increases susceptibility to reinjury.

Genetics

Everyone is born with a pedigree that leads to certain structural anomalies or systemic deficiencies. (I suppose genetics are the ultimate predisposition we all have.) If connective tissue is shorter or longer than normal, you're more vulnerable to sprains, tears, and snaps. Some people have genetic indicators for arthritis, heart disease, obesity, or pain, and there are plenty who

JOINT DISCUSSION
Pitch Perfect

The throwing motion—forward acceleration of the shoulder—is thought to be one of the most "violent" movements in sport, and it can take its toll as it tends to overwork, over-tighten, and overstrengthen the front of the shoulder and, more important, place tremendous strain on the back end of the shoulder. The rear rotator cuff is responsible for decelerating the arm: That is, the arm goes forward rapidly, and as the rear rotator cuff puts on the brakes, it tends to fatigue, weaken, and loosen up a little, which increases the risk of shoulder problems.

To reduce the risk of shoulder or other frame-part injury as well as improve performance, baseball pitchers need to learn proper throwing mechanics at an early age, something we have learned from pioneers like Dr. James Andrews and top-notch therapist Kevin Wilk. In their biomechanics lab at the American Sports Institute in Birmingham, Alabama, they discovered that biomechanical parameters at the instant of foot contact are directly associated with those at the shoulder level. They have helped pinpoint the full kinetic chain from the ground to ball release at the hand. They recommend that young pitchers use a change-up as a safe secondary pitch to complement the fastball, and that they should not add a curveball or slider until they've mastered the mechanics of those first two pitches and their skeletons have matured enough to handle those added stresses, usually around age 14. Their research has shed tremendous light on shoulder function and preventive programs for maintaining a healthy shoulder even in high-performance, overuse-prone situations.

Pitchers must also "exercise" special care at the start of a new season. A multicenter study (presented at the 2010 annual meeting of the American Academy of Orthopaedic Surgeons) showed that in-season, throwing-related injuries to professional pitchers requiring surgery could be traced to *preseason* weakness identified in the external rotators and supraspinatus muscle of the rotator cuff. *(continued)*

haven't been given a fair complement of athletic prowess. When it comes to shoulders, all of this must be taken into account. (This is where "management" comes to the fore.) The best advice I can give is to choose your parents wisely; short of that, remember that your genetics may be the hand you are dealt, but as any good poker player will tell you, it's also how you play the cards. I am one who believes that it is never too late to change your fate.

AND ANOTHER THING . . . OR TWO

Before moving on to the next step, which addresses balky and damaged shoulders, allow me to address a couple of areas that will help you avoid injury and maximize the benefits of a shoulder exercise program.

Posture

Loss of an erect frame is insidious: The decline is imperceptible as it progresses. Each incremental bend or slouch doesn't show up on our radar, but we get the (startling) picture one day when we catch ourselves in a mirror and the image doesn't jibe with the one we have in our memory.

Posture is something you can do a lot about. Rounded shoulders are out, as is lying in bed with your chin near your chest. Some people are never positioned properly, whether they're standing, walking, or sitting, and almost everyone can do something to improve posture. No matter how old you are, these simple tips are worth heeding:

- **Sit up straight,** as parents and teachers constantly harp: head erect and shoulders back—and tighten your abs
- **Stand up straight:** head erect, feet apart at shoulder width, shoulders in line with ankles
- **Walk erect:** head up, shoulders back

De-Stress Your Shoulders

Prolonged sitting at work or when you travel can wreak havoc on your neck and shoul-

To check your posture, stand as you naturally do, sideways in front of a mirror. If your shoulders extend beyond your buttocks, your back is too tight; if the middle of your back is out farther than your buttocks, or if your shoulders and upper body are out in front of your pelvis, you're slumping. Both conditions add unnecessary stress to your knees and your entire frame.

ders. Get up and move around for a couple of minutes every hour. Also, roll your shoulders upward and backward as you pull them back and squeeze your shoulder blades toward each other, as if you were trying to pinch something between them. Try reaching for the sky when you take a break, and move about to keep your frame oiled. Remember, *motion is lotion,* and as one of my very active elderly patients said, "If you rest, you rust."

"De-Sudden" Your Movement

Unless required for sport or self-preservation, abrupt lifts, twists, turns, starts, and stops should be avoided, especially if you are not used to them or not adequately warmed up.

Take a Load Off

Remind yourself often that your body is not a crane. When you pick up anything—free weight or feather—from the floor, bend at the knees, be square to the object, and balance it and yourself as you rise at a measured pace; when you walk with a heavy object, make sure the weight is held close to your body so it is transferred to your heels, not to your toes or the middle of your feet. Be very careful lifting over your head, especially with heavy or awkwardly bulky objects (e.g., loading the almost-full overhead bin on an airplane with your "never should have been allowed on the plane in the first place" carry-on).

Rise Right

Joints, especially older ones, are stiffest first thing in the morning. Don't ask your body parts to do their thing before they've had their coffee, so to speak. Again, no sudden movements upon awakening, and no strenuous activity before you've had a chance to limber up a bit (a Step 4 topic).

RISK AND REWARD

The most important thing to take away from this step is that the muscles, and their associated tendons, can be *worked*. Take action and fine-tune yours, and you'll have taken another broad step toward an active life.

Weak links, together with repetitive wear and tear, prey upon your shoulders. Cartilage is damaged or lost, weakness and imbalances set in, and other soft tissue loses elasticity (just as old rubber bands do), making your inherently unstable shoulders more so. If you take action to strengthen your weak links as best you can (three guesses about how that can be done would likely include exercise, wouldn't they?), you'll be as active as you can be.

Let me repeat: Sedentary is not an option.

And regular golf or tennis or aerobics or circuit training isn't enough, either. If you want to stay healthy or recover faster and more completely from shoulder injury and pain, there's no substitute for building up muscle and fine-tuning coordination with the comprehensive cross-training and support recommendations in the pages that follow.

SORROWFUL SHOULDERS

If you have discomfort or pain in your shoulder, the cause of your ache may actually be originating in a different part of your frame, as we discussed at some length in the knee and lower-back books that preceded this one. Arthritis in the hip or sciatica in the lower back can, via nerve pathways, refer pain to the knee area and masquerade as a knee problem. A sore hip or lower back can also induce an unnatural frame-part alignment to compensate for knee pain; the resulting unnatural biomechanics can cause extra friction and torque on the knee, leading to more pain there. Similarly, unbalanced, tight trapezius muscles; a cervical disk problem; or a pinched nerve that refers pain or weakens the shoulder could be the cause of its discomfort or pain.

Doctors connect the dots to find the source of pain everywhere in the body. A pinched forearm nerve can mimic carpal tunnel symptoms, a damaged brachial plexus (the bundle of nerves deep within the shoulder that acts as a sort of transportation terminal for coming and going brain signals) can show up with shoulder, elbow, or hand symptoms—the list goes on and on. Frame-Work is always about the total body—no matter what the ailment is, parts connected to the affected one must be checked, if for no other reason than to eliminate them from the clinical picture.

IS IT INJURY . . . OR PAIN?

A thorough shoulder examination, including a detailed history, a physical, and appropriate x-rays or imaging studies (when and if needed) will determine if a complaint can be explained simply by the shoulder's inherent mobility (at the expense of stability—remember?) and its susceptibility to overuse. In other words, if a repetitive activity, such as hanging wallpaper or playing an intense tennis match after a long layoff, is the culprit, and the case at hand is a matter of pain that is coming from over-stressed frame parts and inflammation, not serious injury. In these cases, the first prescription is to use the RICE first-aid protocol:

- **Rest:** Take a break from the activity that caused the discomfort. Try to avoid using the shoulder in its "painful arc" (the part of the motion arc that produces significant pain). But don't totally rest a sore shoulder too long, as it has a tendency to freeze up and get very stiff (more on that later). So "relative rest" is a better term.

- **Ice:** Use cold packs for 20 minutes at a time, several times a day. *Do not apply ice directly to the skin.* This is especially true for freezer gel packs that get as cold as your freezer and can cause frostbite on the skin. I prefer a thin washcloth moistened with cool water and wrung out, with the ice or gel pack over that and held in place with an elastic wrap or just draped over the shoulder. A bag of frozen peas or corn can also work nicely (but don't eat them after you've thawed and refrozen them). It is important to note that ice therapy doesn't have to be a chore; you can often apply the ice pack, hold it in place with an Ace wrap, and be up and about.

- **Compression:** An elastic wrap can sometimes improve comfort and also assures maximum effectiveness of the cold therapy. *Do not wrap too tight.* There is a relatively inexpensive product, ThermoActive, that is terrific for shoulders (also knees, ankles, and more): It is a support (actually a circumferential compression therapy system) that fits nicely and is easily applied. It has a removable gel that can be used cold (via freezer) or hot (via microwave), and also an innovative pump that applies compression (www.thermoactive.net). Nursing a sore shoulder has never been easier.

- **Elevation:** To prevent or reduce swelling, do not recline all the way down when you rest, and always keep your shoulder higher than your midsection or core. Prop yourself up on a few pillows and try to avoid sleeping on the affected side.

If necessary, you can use nonsteroidal anti-inflammatory drugs such as aspirin and ibuprofen in conjunction with the above protocol. This course will resolve discomfort/pain issues in most milder cases of shoulder overuse. It will not, however, do a thing when it comes to producing the lotion required for its smooth operation—and resistance to breakdown—after initial recovery. *Motion* supplies that.

But you already knew that, right?

Unfortunately, the first inclination most people have when they've got a sore shoulder is to baby it. As a result, inflammation sticks around longer than it has to, stiffness is more than it should be, and those wonderful muscles we discussed in the last step get out of shape. What was true for the back and the knee is also true for the shoulder: In most cases, the sooner you move it, the sooner you heal it.

As soon as your pain is under control (i.e., you don't feel it when at rest), the recovery and rehabilitation exercises in Step 5 will reduce the time it takes to move from woe to "go" and minimize your susceptibility to a relapse. Slight or even moderate discomfort while you do rehab exercises can occur; if that dissipates quickly afterward, it's an example of pain leading to gain. If it doesn't, either you're doing something wrong or too soon, or something was missed in your workup. Regardless, *stop whatever you're doing and get thee to a doctor.*

Pain is one thing, injury quite another. If your shoulder pain is unremitting, if you have pain at night, if you have experienced dramatic loss of motion and/or strength or can't raise your arm, or if you have chills or fever or sudden weight loss, something might be terribly wrong and you are in need of *immediate* medical attention. After your condition is under control, discuss the recovery program

JOINT DISCUSSION

Shoulder "clicking" is a complaint I hear often from my patients. Most of the time it's nothing to worry about, as it is not all that uncommon for the scapula to "snap" against a rib, or for a tendon to click deeper in the shoulder. Sometimes the bursa in the shoulder will crackle a little. If there is no pain associated with it and/or it is similar in the opposite shoulder, there is usually no need for further investigation.

On the other hand, if pain or a "catching" sensation occurs, you can be sure I'll be putting my trusty detective hat on, looking for deeper problems in the biceps tendon, rotator cuff, or labrum.

in Step 5 with your doctor for possible inclusion in the treatment that follows.

THE INCREDIBLE ARTHROSCOPE

I went on at some length in the knee book about the evolution of this marvel of medical technology that we surgeons are so fond of. These are the two most critical points I made.

- The arthroscope tends to be overused. It's true that it is relatively easy to use and minimally invasive, but it is also true that its effectiveness in treating some conditions, especially arthritis, is far from certain. I'll say it again: A comprehensive examination and evaluation must precede any surgical procedure. In most cases, a more conservative, nonsurgical approach is warranted, including a good rehabilitation program, much of which can be done at home, and this will get easier for patients with a wide variety of musculoskeletal ailments thanks to emerging interactive technologies utilizing gaming platforms (like the Kinect for Xbox or Wii) found in most homes. (More on that later.)

- The arthroscope can be a diagnostic tool as much as a surgical one. MRIs and other scans are terrific, but at best they are only 95 percent accurate, and in some cases a definitive diagnosis can be made only after going in to "scope" things out. Sometimes we look around and find advanced arthritis or another condition that is beyond the scope's repair capability right now. (This news doesn't square with the usual patient expectation that we can fix anything. It isn't always easy for me to discuss this with my patients, but there are some things that they just have to know.)

The good news here is that the scope is being used more and more for shoulder complaints, and most of the ailments that required major open procedures and longer hospital stays when I was in training are now being done through the scope as outpatient procedures. Short of a complete joint replacement (yes, sports fans, it's coming to more operating "theaters" every day), surgeons are doing almost everything else through that marvel of minimally invasive medical technology.

The bad news is that postoperative pain

SHOULDER THIS

The arthroscope is the tool of the devil.
—Dr. Joe Torg

from shoulder procedures usually lasts longer than that for similar arthroscopic procedures in the knee. I'm telling you, I've seen many a patient go home after surgery and complain for weeks and even months about discomfort and difficulty avoiding it. It's hard to get comfortable, especially at night, after shoulder surgery. Some of my "toughest" patients have breezed through knee surgeries but struggled when their shoulders needed repair. This has improved significantly as we have become more aware of the importance of pain management in optimizing patient recovery and outcomes. I suppose the reason pain lingers longer in shoulder cases has to do with the innervation (internal nerve mechanisms) of

JOINT DISCUSSION

My good friend Arnold Schwarzenegger pushed his body to the limit and beyond as a high-level athlete and world-champion bodybuilder. His frame took a beating at times. In terms of medical procedures, he's had more than his share, including heart surgery, knee surgery, and hip replacement surgery. Take it from me: His on-screen persona isn't all make-believe, and he's as tough as they come.

Arnold told me (and I've heard this over and over from other orthopaedic frequent fliers) that nothing was quite like the recovery from rotator cuff surgery. The Terminator himself said he had significant pain, found it hard to get comfortable in the weeks following surgery, and couldn't sleep at night: He had to be propped up and immobile in bed to find any relief. I remember counseling him during his recovery when his deltoid strength returned and he could raise his arm but he didn't have enough strength for external rotation. As usual with Arnold, he worked hard to get back to 100 percent and continues his commitment to personal health, well-being, and fitness, not just for himself but as a matter of national policy.

There are many things we doctors can do to help after every shoulder procedure, but we just haven't yet found a way to maximize comfort and accelerate healing and recovery as much as we'd like. Right now time is a huge ally—it makes the pain go away, and it dulls the memory so that a "total recall" isn't nearly as traumatic as the initial experience was.

the deeper structures, and possibly that we use the joint in different ways than we do the knee, which results in more micromotion and pulling on internal stitches—more irritation to more parts more often.

THE COMPLAINT DEPARTMENT

If you don't manage the initial episodes of shoulder pain related to overuse, or you ignore them altogether when they persist and gut it out when you have to do something involving your shoulders, sooner or later you'll end up on the other side of the pain-injury equation. That's when you'll show up in an office just like mine and get an official diagnosis, and it wouldn't surprise me one bit if what you have is the first of the several complaints that follow.

Impingement Syndrome

There is a whole lot of rubbing and rotation going on in your shoulder when it moves as designed, especially through full abduction— that is, when you move your arms out and away from your body. When the limit is stretched too often or too severely, or shoulder parts are overworked over time, bursitis, tendinitis, or even a small rotator cuff tear (discussed below) can result. Discomfort or

pain, usually centered in the upper part of the shoulder or arm, is the eventual result, and it's not all that uncommon for the ache to interfere with sleep.

Pain forces compromises to make it go away, and those usually result in an imbalance that causes another ailment later on. For example, instead of using the entire shoulder for full arm abduction, the scapula and trapezius compensate and are used to get it up, and the neck area gets strained. I can't tell you how many times I've traced neck and arm pain to shoulder impingement and the stresses it causes. And vice versa. Let's just say that the neck and shoulder are intimately related, for better or for worse.

Excessive pressure can also cause brachial plexopathy, which is characterized by significant inflammation of the brachial plexus nerve bundle deep in the shoulder. Symptoms that can accompany this condition include a tingling or burning sensation in the shoulder; numbness in the shoulder, arm, or hand; weakness of the shoulder; and otherwise

JOINT DISCUSSION

I think a good shoulder specialist needs to be a bit of a neurologist and a vascular man (or woman), too, because shoulder problems are often nerve and/or circulatory problems. An MRI is only one of a host of tests that should be considered for shoulder pain. Others include electromyography (EMG), which assesses electrical activity in muscles; nerve conduction velocity (NCV), which assesses the speed of electrical signals; and multiple standard x-rays. Getting a clear picture in tricky shoulder cases is indeed like putting a large puzzle together.

Extensive testing, however, is the bane of many shoulder specialists' existence. After all, "specialist" usually means "surgeon," and surgeons are like fighter pilots—their whole mission is to "fly" with some fancy high-tech instruments. Most shoulder specialists I know want patients with "good" shoulder problems, the kind that get better with shoulder rehab or, better yet, an operation. Cervical disks and nerve bundles are outside their main area of focus, and they prefer not to devote their limited time and energy to more complex neck and other nonshoulder problems that require physical therapy and other approaches (like, ahem, FrameWork).

The bottom line is shoulder pain often isn't just shoulder pain. When a patient calls and reports shoulder pain, in my mind I go through anything that could explain it, from a torn rotator cuff to a pinched nerve in the neck to a pulmonary lesion or even a heart attack. I quickly ask a series of questions about the pain: What may have caused it? When does it happen? What provokes it? What irritates it? When does it go away? Do you have it at night?

When I see them in my office, I usually tell patients that surgery is down the list I'll be checking off. I inform them about a range of tests from finger strength to reflexes to high-tech scans that will be part of the exam, and that referrals to specialists, including those fighter pilots, may be part of the treatment course. Again, most shoulder problems will get better without surgery, but if you need surgery, the time has never been better.

unexplained deep shoulder-area pain. Tightness and/or impingement can also cause thoracic outlet syndrome, characterized by abnormal pressure on the brachial artery (the main vascular pipeline to the arm), which can also present these symptoms.

The point here is that a doctor must be an excellent diagnostician. Is it carpal tunnel or a pinched neck nerve? Is it brachial plexopathy? A lopsided trapezius? Could it be thoracic outlet syndrome, or is it some combination? To complicate matters further, there isn't a single definitive test for some conditions, including brachial plexopathy and thoracic outlet syndrome. The only way to go is a thorough physical and workup that, yes, will usually include an MRI that helps complete the picture. Sometimes even nerve-conduction studies are needed to see if there is neural contribution to the pain.

Treatment

If you intervene early on, impingement syndrome is easy to address. Cut back or cease altogether the shoulder activity that is causing abnormal stress and use the RICE protocol as often as necessary. As soon as you don't have pain with normal shoulder use, you will need to restore balance to your shoulder, so get

started on the recovery program in Step 5— it's your best bet for avoiding a recurrence.

Frozen-Shoulder Syndrome

First cousin to impingement syndrome is this condition that is officially called adhesive capsulitis (as if we needed yet another -itis). It doesn't mean you wake up one morning with a shoulder that doesn't move; instead, it refers to the gradual loss of the range of shoulder motion. Diminished movement is so gradual, patients often don't even realize when they've lost 50 percent of the range they started with. The scapula and shoulder compensate, masking the motion and function loss. Eventually, tightness and stiffness make even simple arm movements difficult.

There are usually three phases to this complaint, in the order below, that can take from 6 months to more than 2 years to unfold:

- **"Freezing"**: Pain and stiffness build gradually and cause progressive loss of motion.
- **"Thawing"**: Pain diminishes and moving the arm becomes more comfortable, but its range is still limited.
- **"Frozen"**: Some range of shoulder motion returns, but not to its original level.

We don't yet know if this complaint has a

primary cause, but, as we will see in much of this chapter, inflammation plays a starring role. In this case, it tightens the space between the shoulder capsule and the humeral head, which impedes movement.

Frozen shoulder usually affects people between the ages of 40 and 60, and women are more prone to get it. People with diabetes are also at increased risk (and if a diabetic has one frozen shoulder, chances are 50-50 that he or she will have two), along with those who have Parkinson's disease, hyperthyroidism, or cardiovascular disease. But it can happen to anyone (even after breast surgery or an unrelated arm injury), and it can seem as if a severe loss of range happened spontaneously.

Treatment

A frozen shoulder sometimes gets better on its own over time; far more often, it takes months of regular therapy that incorporates moist heat with gentle exercises *three or four times daily,* along with the prudent use of ibuprofen, to get past the discomfort that may be associated with restoring motion and recovery. If pain is severe, you may get a cortisone injection (discussed in the next section). If the condition doesn't improve after several months, your doctor might recom-

mend "going in" with an arthroscope to see if something that didn't show up on any scans is there. At that point the scope can be used to expand the tight shoulder capsule and release scar tissue or adhesions, and the shoulder can be manipulated while the patient is under anesthesia to regain the lost motion and break up any residual adhesions and contractures. And then right back to therapy. Some surgeons also prescribe a CPM (continuous passive motion) machine to keep things moving so that the deep freeze doesn't set back in.

Arthritis, Tendinitis, and Bursitis

The multidirectional mobility of the shoulder results in constant rubbing, rolling, and expansion/contraction of its soft-tissue components. The result of such movement?

Friction.

Which isn't always a bad thing.

Friction causes irritation, which causes inflammation, which causes pain. But friction also helps us stop our automobiles and warm our skin when it is rubbed, among countless other benefits. When it comes to your shoulders, friction lets us know parts are being worked and lets us know when their limits are being challenged. Healthy shoulders keep the irritation associated with movement localized and to a minimum, which, in turn, keeps irritations short term—if they are noticed at all. In biomechanical terms, healthy shoulders transfer and absorb forces efficiently.

As we discussed above, some occupations and recreational interests lead to overuse, and that is a setup for an -itis condition. Of particular import to a fast-growing group of aging baby boomers and seniors, as well as what we now refer to as "mature athletes," age is also a setup, because no matter how carefully one uses one's shoulders, normal friction will take its toll on the soft tissues. Most of us will have to deal with at least one of the three inflammatory shoulder ailments below in our lifetime; the more unfortunate among us will jump from one to another and back. If you've got more than one of these at the same time, my heart goes out to you.

Arthritis

The shoulder actually has two separate joints, the glenohumeral joint (main ball and socket) and the acromioclavicular—or AC—joint (the small joint at the end of the collarbone, where it connects to the acromium of the scapula, just above the ball and socket). Either or both joints can develop arthritis.

The primary symptom of arthritis is deep-seated pain that progressively worsens. As a result of wear and tear, articular (or hyaline) cartilage—that opaque white stuff on the ends of bones that cushions movement—is prone to chondral defects (potholes, I call them) and loose bodies ("chips") that compromise smooth motion and increase friction. The painful inflammation that results from this and/or from other parts that have gotten overrubbed or overstretched is called osteoarthritis (OA). Inflammation escalates as time goes on in just about every case, because who among us can stop using his or her shoulders? Stiffness and loss of shoulder motion and mobility then set in, and it's downhill from there.

Shoulder inflammation flare-ups of any kind usually respond to the first aid described above; when pain is your companion every day and even the simplest tasks are compromised, when over-the-counter (OTC) medications no longer work (or you are taking them like breath mints), you probably have a full-blown case of arthritis and are in a vicious cycle of pain caused by inflammation, restricted movement, more inflammation (because there's no lotion to hasten its exit), more pain, and more restricted movement.

Unless a pothole, a chip, or a tear in the

labrum, rotator cuff, or tendon tissue (discussed below) is a part of the clinical picture, you most likely won't be getting arthroscopic surgery for arthritis. Contrary to the magic-pill temperament most of America has, using the scope to snip here and stitch there isn't always the miracle cure these issues demand. In many cases it plays but a minor role, and in many other cases it wouldn't do any good at all. That's not what a majority of patients want to hear, but I know only one way to practice medicine: Use whatever will *work* in a particular case.

That doesn't mean that a scope is completely out of the question, but the more advanced your arthritis is, the less likely a scope will offer significant, lasting relief. Talk to your surgeon about this very issue and you won't be one of the many disappointed folks who go through a scope procedure only to find that it didn't help the way you thought it would.

A second, less common type of arthritis is rheumatoid arthritis (RA), an autoimmune disease that can affect multiple joints and produce symptoms that are similar to OA. This complaint usually presents at an earlier age; whereas OA is usually diagnosed long after one reaches 40 years of age, RA is com-monly diagnosed in those who have just turned 30. Continuing the theme that women often have more orthopaedic problems than men, women are three times more likely to have RA than men are.

Last but not least, post-traumatic arthritis can present after a traumatic shoulder injury (a dislocation, separation, or fracture, which are discussed below) or as a complication of another injury, such as a labrum tear (keep reading) or a chronic larger rotator cuff tear (called rotator cuff arthropathy). Also, it is not uncommon for the arthritic process to take several years to unfold and become symptomatic. (Readers of the previous book already know that's what happened in my knee.)

Treatment

Treatment of RA is beyond the scope of this book and requires the direction of a physician who treats it on a regular basis. As for the other types of arthritis, the only way I will know how to proceed is to do a thorough examination that includes a thorough history, a physical exam, and multiple x-ray views (sometimes along with MRI, nerve-conduction, and circulation studies if indicated). I want to know about bone alignment, bone quality, soft-tissue swelling, and bone spacing (or, put another way, how much cartilage has been lost), which is critical before I start cutting into a joint. Also, I need to do an assessment of other associated shoulder or neck issues that may be contributing to the dysfunction and pain. This is a process of elimination, a "differential diagnosis" that doctors use to be sure of what is going on before doing anything. If advanced arthritis is the main issue, then the scope shouldn't be used unless a defect, loose body, or tear is also causing some really significant mechanical impingement.

As discussed in the knee book, chondral defects may be repaired using space-age resurfacing techniques. Those still require an open procedure with a 6- to 18-month recovery, but things are evolving every day. Such resurfacing isn't as far along in the shoulder, but it's catching up fast—it's now possible to regenerate focal areas of articular cartilage or joint cushion with techniques like microfracture and autologous chondrocyte transplantation (ACI). As we wait for further advances in that arena, arthroscopic procedures are being used for debridement (clean-out), removal of loose bodies, and repair of other shoulder parts that may be contributing significantly to pain, inflammation, and dysfunction (discussed below).

When prospects for surgical correction aren't favorable, other treatment options for arthritis are available to you and your doctor:

■ Careful use of OTC anti-inflammatory meds

JOINT DISCUSSION
"Tweeners"

I have many patients who, because of their degree of arthritis, are beyond where I can help them with a scope but are not yet to the point that they need or want a shoulder replacement. I call them "tweeners," and there's no shortage of them. We certainly could use more stepwise surgical procedures or other new treatments for arthritis, because it is a huge leap from a simple scope to a major joint replacement. Fortunately, there is more on the near horizon, so stay tuned!

- Ice packs applied for 20 to 30 minutes up to three times a day (some people get more relief from heat, especially when stiffness is an issue; apply a heating pad set on low for 20 to 30 minutes two or three times a day)

- Supplements (see "OTC Supplement Remedies for Arthritis" for specifics)

- Physical therapy, which includes controlled, monitored therapeutic exercise, ultrasound therapy (gentle vibrations that warm deep tissue to improve bloodflow), and other modalities like H-Wave

- Injections:

  - **Cortisone:** This isn't long-acting, so I'll use it if somebody has a bad flare-up or is going away or has a special occasion and wants to feel better for a week or two. In general, this shouldn't be introduced into a joint more than three times a year, because too much exposure can be damaging to the joint. Think of this steroid as a fire extinguisher, not a long-term solution.

  - **Viscosupplementation:** Formulated from a natural substance that is similar to joint fluid, a single injection can last from 6 to 18 months. It is very safe, and it

SHOULDER THIS

OTC Supplement Remedies for Arthritis

Cosamin DS, a glucosamine and chondroitin sulfate formulation from Nutramax Labs that also has manganese and ascorbate (vitamin C); **Cosamin ASU** (avocado-soybean unsaponifiable), also from Nutramax, which includes glucosamine and chondroitin sulfate as well as green-tea extract; **Zyflamend,** from New Chapter Organics, a combination of anti-inflammatory agents; **Limbrel,** a flavocoxid, anti-inflammatory, and antioxidant "medical food" that requires a prescription; **Pycnogenol** (PCO), also available in pine bark or grape-seed extracts; **ginger; turmeric; L-arginine; cayenne pepper; salicin** (willow bark); **acetyl-L-carnitine; gamma linolenic acid** (GLA); **branched-chain amino acids** (BCAA); **coenzyme Q10; omega-3s; flaxseed**

works at all stages of arthritis (although it is more effective early on). I use it on my knee patients so they can exercise comfortably to lose weight and to train support structures, which leads to more permanent relief when the injection wears off. It is a longer-term solution for arthritis pain. Viscosupplementation is not yet FDA approved for use in the arthritic shoulder (hopefully sometime soon), but there have been favorable scientific studies in the shoulder, hip, and other joints, and many physicians are using it "off label" to help those with arthritis who have not responded to other conservative measures.

Treating arthritis isn't easy, and outcomes are uncertain at best. That's why we are doing everything we can to avoid the condition and mitigate its effects. Recent advances in blood testing for inflammation biomarkers allow us to predict and prevent joint wear, and new, high-resolution, 3-D-type qualitative MRI technology now gives doctors a chance to see joints at the metabolic level, which enables us to catch joint surface damage and arthritis at a much earlier stage. But no matter what stage you're in, when pain subsides, do everything *you* can to combat inflammation and break the arthritis cycle: Lose weight, eat right, take supplements, and (oh no, not again!) exercise to improve your prospects for staying active.

Tendinitis

A fraying tendon brings on inflammation, your relentless enemy. Anyone who uses a shoulder repetitively and older people who jump into an activity or intense training program are especially susceptible to tendon microtears that can be quite painful. Age—another relentless enemy—is sometimes the sole explanation for tendinitis, as the supraspinatus muscle is always between a rock and a hard place (the acromion and the humeral head) and gets pinched during normal movement, especially during overhead activities.

Interestingly, tendinitis pain often goes away if the tendon separates from bone or muscle or breaks into two pieces, because, like a rope rubbing hard on the edge of a cliff and snapping, it stops pulling. This is especially true of the biceps tendon in the front of the shoulder. If you can't live with it that way, doctors might be able to stitch it back together; I'd rather treat the tendon when it

JOINT DISCUSSION

If you tear a biceps tendon, you might end up with a bulging biceps, a "Popeye muscle." One of my patients, a police officer, really liked the way his looked when he wore short sleeves and didn't think getting a "gun" like that on his other arm would be so bad.

first starts to tear, whether it is the biceps or the rotator cuff tendon, just as I prefer treating a small separation in a pant seam before it rips open altogether.

As tears recur and are more chronic, the tendon shows less and less inflammation and more signs of internal damage, and a type of avascular (and thus with limited healing ability) scar tissue forms, which we call tendinopathy. Unless the aggravating activity is stopped for a sufficient amount of time, the tendon will never heal completely.

Treatment

Most tendinitis cases are treated conservatively to give the body a chance to heal itself. A combination of anti-inflammatory medications, physical therapy, and shoulder-stretching and -strengthening exercises usually does the trick, especially if they are used early on.

If the condition doesn't improve over time (up to a year is appropriate in most cases), outpatient surgery to remove unhealthy tendon tissue may be recommended. Tendon repair can be accomplished with arthroscopic techniques in most cases, although sometimes open procedures are still required. Newer technologies such as biologic scaffolds and cell therapies, including PRP (protein-rich plasma), are being utilized to enhance and accelerate healing in and around the shoulder, but more research is needed in that regard. I am a big believer in the potential of these new-age treatments, but we are not quite there yet. For most surgical shoulder repairs, recovery and rehab can take up to 6 months before a return to full activities is possible.

As always, the best treatment is prevention. Condition your shoulder for repetitive activity with stretching, warmup (including a hot shower or bath, or a moist heating pad as necessary), and the directed exercises in Step 5. Just as important, increase repetitions gradually to forestall the inflammation that arises from overuse, and allow adequate recovery after exercise or shoulder use/overuse.

Bursitis

This complaint is marked by inflammation (there it is again!) of the bursa, the lubricating sac located just over the rotator cuff. Way back when I was a resident, before we had a firm hold on shoulder biomechanics and functional anatomy, any pain associated with raising an arm was called bursitis; we know better today and favor a much more specific anatomic diagnosis, but this is still a condition that causes shoulder pain for millions of people.

Bursa inflammation is usually a case of "where there's smoke, there's fire." That is, the swelling isn't caused by something going on within the bursa; instead, labrum, rotator cuff, or biceps irritation or tear—or a combination of these—may be the culprit.

Treatment

This complaint, along with the two other -itis ones above, is closely linked with impingement syndrome. In the unlikely event that there aren't any issues with another shoulder part that should be addressed first (as discussed below), the recommended treatment is the first approach for treating impingement: RICE and rest. If bursa swelling persists in the absence of other major shoulder issues, a cortisone shot will often do the trick, followed by some rehab and other preventive measures.

Subluxation and Dislocation

The ball-on-a-tee glenohumeral joint is front and center here both for those born with extra mobility in the inherently mobile shoulder joint and for those who overuse it. They are the primary candidates for this "popping out" malady that also afflicts plenty who aren't in either category.

If the shoulder partially pops out, it is called a subluxation; if it's out all the way, it's a full-blown dislocation. As discussed earlier, if you experience one subluxation, you are likely to experience another (especially if you are young and/or active, as you should be); if you overstretch soft tissue that holds things together, it usually doesn't return all the way to its original form and strength. It may take years, or even decades, of subluxations before a shoulder is dislocated—stretched all the way out to a point where only a doctor can put it back in.

It can happen a lot sooner, too, and it frequently does as the result of a traumatic blow from a sports collision or from a hard fall that pulls the arm in an extreme direction. The joint can dislocate forward (by far the most common direction for subluxation and dislocation)—an occurrence whereby the upper arm bone is forced out of the front part of the joint—or it can dislocate backward or downward. Some unfortunate folks have multidirectional instability, and that is not a good thing unless you are a circus contortionist. The force of the blow also usually causes tears in ligaments, the labrum, and sometimes even tendons. Subluxations usually pop back on their own, while dislocations will send you screaming for the nearest ER to get put back in place.

Whenever or however it happens, it's a matter of compromised shoulder biomechanics that doctors have learned a lot about in recent years. For example, we now know that subluxations and dislocations can cause tears in the labrum (discussed below) that compromise stability further, which increases the likelihood of another episode. Also, subluxations can be subtle and in throwing athletes cause a "dead arm"-type feeling after a hard throw. If your shoulders and other joints are Gumby-like and superloose, you may have a version of the genetic disorder called Ehlers-Danlos syndrome, in which there is intrinsic pathology with your body's collagen, causing it to be way more elastic than it should be.

Treatment

If you've dislocated your shoulder, get to the emergency room as soon as possible. The doctor will order x-rays to evaluate the extent of the dislocation and rule out a related fracture (also discussed below). Then you'll be mildly sedated so the doctor can push the shoulder joint back into place. Severe pain is relieved immediately after this shoulder reduction procedure. Also, you should always be checked for nerve damage, which fortunately occurs only rarely with a shoulder dislocation.

You'll have to rest your shoulder for a few weeks and keep it in a sling for a few days. Ice can be used for 20 to 30 minutes a couple of times during the day to relieve soreness and swelling. No surprise, you'll have to exercise, slowly and incrementally, starting with stretches until a full range of motion is restored; then you can move on to resistance exercises that restore shoulder strength—the strength that helps prevent a recurrence. If your shoulder is loose and prone to subluxation and/or dislocation, you will have to modify your exercise routines, especially weight training, to avoid the positions and arc of motion in which the shoulder starts to slip. You can still work the shoulder in the nonvulnerable positions, something that can actually protect against instability.

If you experience multiple dislocations over a couple of years (or recurrent episodes of subluxation), surgery may be necessary to repair torn or stretched ligaments and/or the labrum, if it is torn or separated from the socket, so they are better able to hold the joint in place. (This is especially true for younger active individuals.) In fact, many surgeons are recommending surgery to stabilize the shoulder after the *first* dislocation in younger athletes, which is something that makes tremendous sense. Surgery is now accomplished through the scope as an outpatient procedure in the vast majority of cases. Again, you'll need to keep the shoulder immobilized for a few weeks while undergoing physical therapy. Full recovery requires several months.

Shoulder Separation

When you hear of an athlete getting a shoulder separation, which is sometimes referred to as an AC sprain, the acromioclavicular (AC) joint—where the collarbone (clavicle) connects to a bony knob (acromium process) on the shoulder blade (scapula)—is the focus.

A separation doesn't have to be the result of a tackle on a football field or a collision on an ice rink; taking a tumble off a bicycle or a stoop could do the trick. A mild, or Grade 1, separation overstretches the two AC ligaments and causes the area over the AC joint to be tender, which makes lifting the arm somewhat painful. A Grade 2 separation includes partial tears in one or both AC ligaments accompanied by significantly more pain, and perhaps a slight bump over the AC joint. If you have a Grade 3 separation, your shoulder will be visibly deformed and one or

JOINT DISCUSSION

You don't have to have a dislocation to experience AC joint pain. You can have arthritis of the AC joint and develop a painful prominence over it secondary to spur formation. Also, a rare condition called DCO (distal clavicle osteolysis) can occur. It is more widely referred to as weight lifter's shoulder, and young people who lift heavy weights (especially with bad technique and repetitive overload) without a balanced program are especially prone to getting it. The result is degeneration and loss of the end of the collarbone near the AC joint.

both ligaments are completely torn: The result is an obvious bump.

Treatment

If intense pain does not subside after the injury, or if you see a bump, get it checked by an orthopaedic specialist. X-rays, including "stress views," for which you hold weights at each side (so you have a comparison), will determine the extent of the separation. Grade 3 sprains are pretty obvious and do not usually need the stress views.

Most AC injuries are treated conservatively. You'll probably just wear a sling to immobilize your shoulder for a few days until the pain improves. Icing the shoulder for 20 to 30 minutes two or three times a day will help reduce inflammation and pain. Ibuprofen or other OTC NSAIDs (nonsteroidal anti-inflammatory drugs, which also include aspirin) can be taken as needed during that initial period, too.

Almost instantly, the joint can be put back into motion with physical therapy and/or recovery exercises like the ones in Step 5. Don't be surprised if it takes a month to return to normal activity, however. For contact sports such as ice hockey and football, in which you often lead the way into collisions with the shoulder (with the AC joint at the epicenter of contact), a pad can be used to get you back in action faster and more comfortably.

Surgery is being used less and less for AC joint injuries, even for complete tears. Most can be managed conservatively, especially in the acute phase. If symptoms persist on a more chronic basis, surgery can always be done to improve the situation. Surgery is sometimes recommended from a cosmetic standpoint, especially in women who wear gowns regularly and put a premium on shoulder symmetry. Also, Grade 3 tears in the dominant arm of high-level overhead or throwing athletes deserve surgical consideration, weighing the pros and the cons carefully. If you have surgery, you'll be wearing a sling intermittently for a couple of weeks, and you'll definitely be sent to physical therapy.

Torn Rotator Cuff

Although these muscles can be torn as a result of a single traumatic injury, most tears are the result of repetitive overuse and/or aging and attrition. This injury rose to prominence many years ago when it was diagnosed in a slew of major-league baseball pitchers.

They and high-profile stars in other sports that deliver a heavy pounding to the shoulder had to undergo a major open procedure, and the rehabilitation was arduous and long. Its outcome regarding functional recovery was uncertain at best.

Fortunately, we've come a long way in all areas. We're repairing things now that we never knew had to be repaired. Progress has been driven as much by patients who wanted to stay active and do the things they always did as by the advancements that are sought as a matter of course in every field of medicine. Tools and techniques are greatly improved, recoveries are more tolerable, and outcomes much, much better. Of special import to future advancements is something I mentioned earlier: We know so much more about the biomechanics of the shoulder joint, especially the changes that occur in it as we age. We connected the dots between imbalances, instability, and injury.

While analyzing MRI scans for numerous shoulder injuries, we doctors weren't entirely surprised to discover that a huge percentage of people over 40 have cuff tears that are asymptomatic. We had seen plenty of bulging spinal disks on film in that group that didn't cause discomfort or pain, either. Nonetheless, a rotator cuff tear is a common cause of pain and disability among adults. It occurs most in the supraspinatus muscle, but other parts of the cuff can be involved, too.

Rotator cuff tears usually occur in the dominant shoulder. Some of the signs of a tear include:

- Atrophy or thinning of the muscles about the shoulder

- Pain when lifting the arm

- Pain when lowering the arm from a fully raised position

- Weakness when lifting or rotating the arm

- Crepitus—a crackling sensation when moving the shoulder in certain positions

- Night pain—especially when lying on the involved side

Symptoms of a rotator cuff tear may develop right away after a trauma, such as a lifting injury or a fall on the affected arm. When the tear occurs with an injury, there may be sudden acute pain, a snapping sensation, and an immediate weakness of the arm and inability to raise it overhead. Symptoms may also develop gradually with repetitive overhead activity or following long-term wear. Pain in the shoulder can radiate down the side of the upper arm to the "soldier patch" area (where the stripes on a military uniform are). At first the pain may be mild and present only with overhead activities such as reaching or lifting. It may be relieved by OTC medications such as aspirin or ibuprofen. Over time the pain may become noticeable at rest or with no activity at all. There may be pain when lying on the affected side and at night.

Treatment

Diagnosis of a rotator cuff tear is based on the symptoms, physical examination, and scans. Your doctor will examine the shoulder to see whether it is tender in any specific area or whether there is a deformity. He or she will measure the range of motion of the shoulder in several different directions and will test the strength of the arm in multiple planes with a focus on rotation. The doctor will also check for instability or other problems with the shoulder joint. Plain x-rays of a shoulder with a rotator cuff tear are often normal or only show some spurs around the AC joint. They do not show the cuff or other internal structures; for this reason, the doctor may order an additional study, such as an ultrasound or MRI, that can better visualize cuff tendons and other soft tissue and pinpoint where and how large the tear is. Size does matter in terms of cuff tears, and MRI scans can also determine if there are additional problems such as a labral tear, or if there is a massive cuff tear with retraction of the tendon ends, making repair more complicated.

In many instances, nonsurgical treatment can provide pain relief and can improve the function of the shoulder. Options may include:

■ Rest and limited overhead activity

■ Use of a sling (not for long, however; shoulders freeze up pretty quickly when injured or painful)

■ Anti-inflammatory medication

■ Steroid injection

■ Strengthening exercise and physical therapy

Your orthopaedic surgeon may recommend surgery if:

■ Nonsurgical treatment does not relieve symptoms

■ The tear is in the shoulder of the dominant arm of an active person

■ Maximum strength in the arm is needed for overhead work or sports

Many surgical repairs can be done on an outpatient basis. In general, three approaches are available:

■ **Arthroscopic Repair:** In most cases, small, pencil-size instruments are inserted through tiny incisions instead of a large incision to close and repair tears, and/or to shave bone that impinges upon shoulder function.

■ **Mini-Open Repair:** Newer techniques and instruments allow surgeons to perform a complete rotator cuff repair through a small incision, typically 4 to 6 centimeters. Sometimes arthroscopic procedures are combined with mini-open technique.

■ **Open Surgical Repair:** A traditional open surgical incision is often required if the tear is large or complex or if additional reconstruction, such as a tendon transfer, has to be done. In some severe cases, in which arthritis has developed, one option is to replace the shoulder joint (discussed below).

The type of surgery performed depends on the size, shape, and location of the tear. A partial tear (i.e., not full thickness) may require only a trimming or smoothing procedure, called a debridement, and probably removal of overlying impinging bone. A complete tear within the thickest part of the tendon is repaired by suturing the two sides of the tendon back together. If the tendon is torn away from where it inserts into the bone of the arm (humerus), it is repaired and reattached directly to bone using mini-suture anchors delivered through the scope.

In the operating room, your surgeon may remove part of the acromion, the front portion of the scapula, as part of the procedure if it is impinging on the tendon and contributing to the tear. Other conditions related to bone abnormalities, such as arthritis of the AC joint or a torn biceps tendon or labrum, may also be addressed.

The affected arm is immobilized after surgery to allow the tear to heal. The length of immobilization depends upon the severity of the tear and the quality of the tissue that was repaired. The weaker and more beat-up the tissue, the more cautious one needs to be post-op. These issues are best determined by your surgeon. A strong commitment to rehabilitation is important to achieve a good surgical outcome. As always, an exercise program (Step 5) will help regain motion and strength in the shoulder. It begins with passive motion and advances to active and resistive exercises. Complete recovery will take several months, or more in some cases. The doctor will examine the outcome to advise when it is safe to return to overhead work and sports activity.

Labrum Tear

Sports injuries, falls, and other traumatic injuries, as well as the overuse most of us are prone to at one time or another, can cause tears to the doughnut of rubbery material that crowns the glenoid. It buffers the space between the ball and socket and gets compressed with every shoulder movement. Squeeze it violently enough or rub it often enough, and it'll begin to fray or come apart. It doesn't take much sometimes—a sudden pull, as when you try to lift a heavy object, is enough to do the trick.

Five or more decades of normal living take their toll, too. It's more than likely you have at least a small tear if you're a boomer or older, but just as likely that it's asymptomatic. Our bodies tend to accommodate a sometimes stiff shoulder and its minor creaks. In addition to constant or significant pain, symptoms when something is really wrong in your labrum are similar to those associated with a torn rotator cuff:

- Catching, locking, popping, or grinding
- Occasional night pain or pain with daily activities
- A sense of instability in the shoulder
- Decreased range of motion
- Loss of strength

When a tear causes pain and compromises normal movement—whether that's painting a ceiling or throwing a baseball—we doctors are on the case.

Treatment

Your doctor will take a history of your injury and ask if you remember a specific incident or if the pain gradually increased. He or she will do several physical tests to check range of motion, stability, and pain. X-rays do not reveal soft-tissue tears, but they will be ordered to see if there are reasons other than a torn labrum for your problems. For an assessment of that, the doctor may order a computed tomography (CT) scan or a magnetic resonance imaging (MRI) scan. In both instances, a contrast medium may be injected into the joint before the MRI is performed (called MR arthrography) to help detect tears. Ultimately, however, the diagnosis may need to be confirmed with arthroscopic surgery.

Tears can be located either above (superior) or below (inferior) the middle of the glenoid socket. A SLAP lesion (superior labrum, anterior [front] to posterior [back]) is a tear of the rim above the middle of the socket that may also involve the biceps tendon. High-level athletes who rely primarily on their shoulder are particularly at risk for that complaint. A tear of the rim below the middle of the glenoid socket that also involves the inferior glenohumeral ligament is called a Bankart lesion and results in instability of the shoulder. As we mentioned above, tears of the glenoid rim often occur with other shoulder injuries, such as a dislocated shoulder (full or partial).

Until the final diagnosis is made, your physician may prescribe anti-inflammatory medication and rest to relieve symptoms. It would be an exception if rehabilitation exercises to rebalance and strengthen the rotator cuff muscles (again, Step 5) were not included in your treatment. The same holds true for some targeted stretching. If these conservative measures are insufficient, your physician may recommend a further workup with imaging studies that ultimately results in a trip to the repair shop for arthroscopic surgery to trim, or even better, repair the labrum and other associated problems.

After surgery, you will need to keep your shoulder in a sling for a few weeks. Your physician will also prescribe gentle, passive, pain-free range-of-motion exercises. When the sling is removed, you will need to do motion and flexibility exercises and gradually

JOINT DISCUSSION

When I was a resident, we never talked about labrum tears. It wasn't even in our vocabulary. Now pretty much everyone has got one—but we doctors have to be careful not to overrate them. I probably have some tearing of my labrum or cuff (lots of miles on me), and you probably do, too, if you are anywhere near my age or older. But I don't plan on offering it up to one of the many superior shoulder guys I know, because I can live with it as it is, thank you very much. Chances are you might be able to live with a labrum tear, especially if you employ the preventive prescriptive throughout this book.

start to strengthen your shoulder. Athletes can usually begin doing sport-specific exercises 6 to 8 weeks after surgery, although it will be 3 to 4 months before the shoulder is fully healed.

Fractures

For a change, overuse doesn't have much to do with broken shoulder bones. Acute trauma, like a hard fall on the outstretched arm or shoulder or a heavy blow, pretty much accounts for every crack we see in the shoulder. For individuals who have weakened bones from osteoporosis, it doesn't take much impact to fracture, or even shatter, the upper arm and shoulder area. The only time overuse is involved in a fracture is in the case of stress fractures that can occur in the upper arm or shoulder, especially in overhead-throwing athletes doing too much too soon, without allowing adequate time for recovery. (I cover stress fractures in much greater detail in *FrameWork: Your 7 Step Program for Healthy Muscles, Bones, and Joints.*) I'll just say that a stress fracture can happen at any age, to Little Leaguers or major leaguers, and even to military recruits, whose shoulders are not accustomed to repetitive overhead activity such as training to throw hand grenades.

The most common site of a fracture is the clavicle, especially for athletes (notably cyclists) and for young children whose bones everywhere have yet to grow to full strength. Fractures can sometimes occur at the head or neck of the upper arm (humerus) where it connects to the shoulder. The elderly, who have weaker bones in general because of the aforesaid osteoporosis, are prone to this injury. Fractures of the shoulder blade (scapula) are rare but can occur as a result of a heavy impact from an auto accident or a fall.

Most shoulder-related fractures are pretty symptomatic, causing severe pain, swelling, and bruising about the clavicle, shoulder, or upper arm. You likely won't be able to lift your arm, and there may be a visible deformity. In addition, there can be numbness down into the arm or hand.

Treatment

Treatment will vary tremendously depending on the type of fracture, the bone involved, and the age of the patient. Some will need only a sling followed by early motion exercises and rehab. Others will require surgery and fixation with plates, screws, or rods. This is best determined by your treating

JOINT DISCUSSION

To elaborate a bit on the shattered clavicle in my youth that I mentioned in the preface, it happened right before football season, but it didn't happen on a playing field. It was the result of clowning around, horseplay with one of my neighborhood buddies, roughing it up, hitting each other—just messing around, as spirited youths are wont to do. I was chasing him in the streets near where we lived, and he grabbed a traffic-light pole and executed a perfect 90-degree turn to elude me. I instantaneously changed my course to coincide with his new one and dove for his midsection.

I hadn't counted on losing my footing.

And I most certainly hadn't counted on becoming personally acquainted with that steel pole, which broke my fall—temporarily, as I was soon writhing in pain on the sidewalk—and demolished my clavicle in the process.

When it comes to kids and their bones, we bone doctors say that if two broken pieces are in the same room, they'll heal really fast and really well. (I suppose the growing process in children compensates somewhat for the injuries that come with their spirited play.) I'm happy to say that was indeed the case with that broken clavicle of my youth. In the interest of full disclosure now, however, I must say that in addition to my missing an entire football season, the prominent bump that appeared on my shoulder shortly after the trauma is still there if I look close enough.

Ah, memories.

orthopaedic surgeon. Anti-inflammatory medication can help control pain until it subsides, but I recommend only a few days of NSAIDs, because studies have suggested that they may extend fracture healing time. Some fractures in adults, such as clavicle fractures, can be very stubborn and heal either very slowly (delayed union) or not at all (nonunion). Sometimes a bone stimulator (a simple, nonpainful device worn for short periods every day) can help turn on the healing process or even accelerate it. Also, as we are always harping on prevention and things you can do to help (or hinder) your healing and recovery, a fracture should be yet another in a long list of wake-up calls to stop smoking, as smoking (including the effects of secondhand smoke) interferes with fracture healing and bone growth.

Once your fracture starts to knit (or if it has been securely stabilized surgically), you can usually begin (here it comes) gentle range-of-motion exercises, followed by strengthening and then a gradual return to

SHOULDER THIS

Fall Prevention

- Avoid shoes with slick soles. (If you just can't pass up a pair, have a cobbler affix textured strips to the soles.)

- Avoid extra-thick soles. (Work boots are great for avoiding the ravages of nails, broken glass, and the like, but they are extra-heavy after wearing them for hours—a setup for tripping going up or down a staircase, or just getting into your truck or SUV.)

- Laced shoes are safer than slip-ons.

- The higher the heel, the greater the risk of falling. (Save the spikes, ladies, for special occasions, preferably in good weather.)

- Long coats, pants, and robes can trip you up.

- Stay well hydrated and don't skip meals— they prevent dizziness. (Heart conditions and some OTC and prescription meds can also make you dizzy, so check with your doctor if you've been tottering enough to notice.)

- Get an annual eye exam and wear your glasses or contacts. Conversely, don't wear reading glasses if you get up to walk around. Also, get regular checkups, especially if there are issues with balance or dizziness.

- Exercise! Weight training to stay strong prevents falls and makes your bones better able to withstand a fall, and tai chi and other exercises (I like the yoga tree pose) improve balance.

- Fall-proof your abode: Get rid of clutter, run power cords around traffic areas, secure throw rugs and area rugs with two-sided tape, have adequate lighting in all traffic areas, clean up spills right away, and use rubber mats in bathrooms.

the activities you enjoy. One last word of advice, especially for women: Your first fracture—anywhere, anytime—should prompt you to find out more about your overall bone health and whether you have osteopenia or osteoporosis. This is especially true if the fracture occurred with relatively minor trauma, and by that I mean anything less than a major motor-vehicle accident or a fall from a very large height. Normal healthy bones are very strong and should not break from trips and falls, whether it's your ankle, hip, or shoulder. Talk to your doctor and get a simple, noninvasive baseline Dexa scan. Also talk about prevention, including calcium, vitamin D, and exercise.

Total Shoulder Degeneration

The 23,000 complete shoulder joint replacements that are performed yearly pale in comparison with the 700,000 knee and hip replacements that are done in the same time frame. The success rates of this relatively new procedure are improving dramatically thanks to newer designs and techniques—they are beginning to rival that of knee and hip replacement—so you can be sure it won't take long for it to be a given. If you have advanced osteoarthritis, rheumatoid arthritis, post-

Chronic steroid use, deep-sea diving, sickle-cell disease, and heavy alcohol use are risk factors for avascular necrosis, to which hips and shoulders are particularly susceptible.

injury arthritis, rotator cuff arthropathy (a combination of severe arthritis and an irreparable tear in a rotator cuff tendon), avascular necrosis (death of bone cells), or a severe fracture, your orthopaedic surgeon will discuss this option with you.

Symptoms that indicate a shoulder replacement may be in a patient's future are similar to those associated with the shoulder complaints discussed above. Patients who have significant arthritis typically describe a deep ache within the shoulder joint associated with loss of motion and mobility in the shoulder. Initially, the pain feels worse with movement and activity, and eases with rest. As the arthritis progresses, the pain may occur even at rest. By the time a patient sees a physician for the shoulder pain, he or she often has pain at night and it may be severe enough to prevent a good night's sleep.

The patient's shoulder may make grinding or grating noises when moved, or the shoulder may catch, grab, clunk, or lock up. Over time, the patient will notice further loss of motion and/or weakness in the affected shoulder. Simple daily activities such as reaching into a cupboard, dressing, toileting, and washing the opposite armpit may become increasingly difficult.

If you're a candidate for a shoulder replacement, your examination x-rays revealed one (and usually more) of the following:

- Loss of the normal space between articular cartilage surfaces
- Flattening or irregularity in the shape of a bone or bones
- Bone spurs
- Loose pieces of bone and cartilage floating inside the joint

Treatment

Patients with bone-on-bone osteoarthritis and intact rotator cuff tendons are generally good candidates for conventional total shoulder replacement, and there are several different types. The usual one involves replacing the arthritic joint surfaces with a highly polished metal ball attached to a stem, and a plastic socket.

Shoulder replacement surgery is performed on an inpatient basis, and most patients are discharged from the hospital on the second or third day after the operation. The components used in the procedure come in various sizes. If the bone is of good quality, your surgeon may choose to use a noncemented or press-fit humeral component. If the bone is soft, the humeral component may be implanted with bone cement. In most cases, an all-plastic glenoid component is implanted with bone cement. Implantation of a glenoid component is not advised if the glenoid has good cartilage, the glenoid bone is severely deficient, or the rotator cuff tendons are irreparably torn. Depending on the condition of the shoulder, your surgeon may replace only the ball. Sometimes this decision is made in the operating room at the time of surgery. Some surgeons replace the ball when it is severely fractured and the socket is normal.

Another type of shoulder replacement is called reverse total shoulder replacement. This surgery was developed in Europe in the 1980s and was approved by the FDA for use in the United States in 2004. Reverse total shoulder replacement is used for people who have:

- Completely torn rotator cuffs and
- The effects of severe arthritis (arthropathy) or
- Had a previous shoulder replacement that failed.

For these individuals, a conventional total shoulder replacement could still leave them with pain and the inability to raise the arm higher than 90 degrees. In a reverse total shoulder replacement, the socket and metal ball are switched: A metal ball is attached to the shoulder bone, and a plastic socket is attached to the upper arm bone.

Patients usually start gentle physical therapy on the first day after the operation, which is part of a well-planned rehabilitation program including home exercises that is critical to the success of a shoulder replacement.

They wear an arm sling during the day for the first several weeks after surgery and wear it at night for 4 to 6 weeks. Most patients are able to perform simple activities such as eating, dressing, and grooming within 2 weeks after surgery. Driving a car is not allowed for 6 weeks, and sports and heavy lifting are usually not recommended for a minimum of 6 months.

One caution before we move on: It's easy to overwork the shoulder after this surgery, because you are finally freed from pain. Follow closely your doctor's recommendations about not overdoing it. Otherwise you might damage your new joint and reduce your chance for optimal recovery.

PRIOR TO SURGERY

You should know a thing or two about some critical factors that influence the outcome of surgery, which I discuss with all my patients

JOINT DISCUSSION

Shoulder replacement surgery is highly technical. It should be performed by a surgical team with experience in this procedure. Each case is unique, and your surgeon will evaluate your situation carefully before making any decisions. Do not hesitate to ask what type of implant will be used in your situation and why that choice is right for you.

before they lie down on the operating table. Right up front in the discussion is the importance of realistic expectations and strict compliance with physical therapy and rehab exercise programs. Other factors on the agenda include:

■ Success is usually determined by the degree of injury or damage. In other words, full recovery may not be possible.

■ Professional and higher-level athletes who have the same injury have better prospects for complete recovery because of highly developed support muscles and conditioning programs. They are also goal oriented and highly motivated to do all the necessary work for optimal recovery.

■ You should return to intense physical activity only under the direction of your surgeon. It is usually a stepwise progression, like advancing to the next level in a video game.

■ Each surgery has a different recovery timetable based on exactly what was done.

■ For all surgeries, the better shape you are in going into it, the quicker your recovery will usually be. (Another reason to be active year-round!)

■ If your job involves heavy work, such as construction labor, you may require more time to return to some or all of your work responsibilities than if you have a sedentary job.

■ Choose your surgeon wisely, and get a second opinion if you are uncertain. Find the shoulder guru in your region (more on that later in the Additional Resources area).

■ Tap into the power of the mind to optimize your recovery. I've seen it over and over again: Attitude fuels outcomes. Stay positive. If there is an abnormal level of anxiety (some manageable anxiety about injury, illness, or surgery is normal) or depression, get properly evaluated by a professional, as these mental-stress-overload conditions have been shown to result in suboptimal results after a wide variety of surgical procedures.

A BALANCED LIFE

Whether they arise from trauma or overuse, sorrowful shoulders can usually be traced to an imbalance between two or more frame parts in and around the shoulder joint: A muscle is overdeveloped here, underdeveloped there; a surface on one side of a gap wears more than the one on the other side; one tendon or ligament loses more tensile strength than another; one bone changes its contour, another doesn't; the posterior capsule is tighter than the anterior capsule. To function at a high level, you have to have the whole megillah working as it was designed to do. (Picture an orchestra working in concert—every instrument is marvelous, but the result would be a mess if one dominated all the time.)

As we discussed earlier, some sports activities generate tremendous forces across the shoulder, accentuating imbalances, and some people play sports aggressively without the proper preventive conditioning or professional training, tempting fate. If your shoulder is injured, you are a prime candidate for other imbalances to develop all over your body.

The immobilization and long recoveries associated with the complaints we've discussed in this step often contribute to imbalance because parts are being used sparingly or not at all. Imbalance is also the result if one does not adhere strictly to a rehab program, or—as I have preached in all of my Frame-Work books—from improperly designed, poorly balanced fitness programs. (Even well-meaning fitness enthusiasts and fitness professionals can create workouts that actually create imbalances in your frame. This is also common with individuals or athletes who favor a single sport or activity and do not

SHOULDER THIS

It ain't the years, it's the miles.

include preventive conditioning to fight the imbalances created by it.) Age, and the accommodations one makes for the wear and tear that comes with it, explain a lot of the shoulder imbalances I see. Many older patients replaced normal movements that had caused discomfort with movement that didn't. That solved the immediate problem, but there were less-than-ideal consequences down the road.

I have said again and again that a surgeon's first goal should be prevention. We are spending more than $1 trillion on health care in the United States, and only about 2 percent of that goes to avoiding treatment of disease and surgical and other invasive procedures. The rest is spent on patchwork after things go wrong. We will never solve out-of-control costs until our focus shifts from being Dr. Fix-Its to being prevention experts. New treatments are fantastic, even magical, but they're expensive and ever more so. (As a nation, we continue to approach the health-care crisis the way we approached Wall Street and the auto industry when they were failing—with a bailout mentality. Wait for it to break, then we can fix it or bail it out.) It might be biting the hand that feeds me, but much better value for our dollars comes from investing in approaches that keep people out of my office. In more ways than one, it seems, it comes down to balance.

Imbalance, like inflammation or injury, is your enemy. As we've discussed at some length, it comes in many varieties but first comes into play as the result of the extremes: constant overuse or a sedentary existence. "Use it or lose it" is never more applicable than when it comes to the shoulder. "Use it" is not, however, about "Just do it"; rather, it is all about "Just do it right." The only way to avoid injuring your shoulder is to use it correctly, and the only way to recover fastest and best from an injury is to move it correctly as soon as possible.

SHOULDER STUDY

The prevention I'm so fond of starts with sober consideration of your general health and overall fitness, and with finding out if you have any of those weak links we discussed in Step 1. Remember, a chain is only as strong as its weakest link, as that's where it is most likely to fail. Same for your frame. After you answer the questions on the following pages, you'll come face-to-face with any muscle imbalances, weakness, atrophy, and/or loss in range of motion *before* you start exercising your shoulders. Most important, you'll find out if you have any red flags—those ticking time bombs we covered in Step 2—that preclude any physical activity until they're resolved with the help of a physician. The focus is the shoulder, but as you'll soon see, shoulder health goes way beyond that ball and socket alone.

In less than 30 minutes, you'll have a snapshot of what kind of shape you're in and what you have to work on. The scoring system I devised for your questionnaire follows the scheme my mechanic uses when he goes over my car. Every aspect of your health as it relates to your shoulders gets a color rating:

- **Green** means smooth sailing.
- **Yellow** means something needs to be watched and/or worked on.
- **Red** means let's do something about it *right now.*

I've used this color-coded approach in my practice for many years with athletes and active individuals, and it gets to the heart of the matter very quickly. Circle the appropriate color for each question that follows (and be brutally honest, or you'll only be cheating yourself). Again, if you circle any "red" responses, be sure to discuss them with your doctor—or better yet, an orthopaedic surgeon or sports medicine specialist—and proceed with caution in Step 5 after he or she gives you the green light to do so.

HISTORY

1. Do you have a family history of significant shoulder problems?

a. No	green
b. Yes	yellow
c. Major shoulder surgery	red

2. Do you ever "baby" your shoulder(s), moving it (or both of them) gingerly to avoid pain or discomfort?

a. No	green
b. Rarely, or after a hard workout	yellow
c. I think of myself as a one-armed bandit	red

3. Does your shoulder "click," "catch," or "pop"?

a. No	green
b. Every now and then	yellow
c. They call me Rice Krispies	red

4. Do you have any stiffness or tightness in your shoulder(s) upon awakening (i.e., until you shower or move around for a while), after sitting still for more than 30 minutes, or for no apparent reason?

a. No	green
b. Only the day after a hard workout	yellow
c. I don't remember when it wasn't stiff	red

5. Do you find that you change your plans or activities (e.g., pass on a tennis date) because of a shoulder problem?

a. No	green
b. Occasionally (no more than a few times a year)	yellow
c. My shoulder is my daily planner	red

6. Do you have difficulty falling asleep at night or awaken during the night because of shoulder discomfort?

a. No	green
b. Rarely, or minor difficulty	yellow
c. I toss and turn like a rotisserie	red

7. Do you have pain while lying on either shoulder at night in bed?

a. No	green
b. Rarely	yellow
c. Almost nightly, tossing and turning to get comfy	red

8. Does low barometric pressure (i.e., damp, rainy weather) make your shoulders ache?

a. No	green
b. Rarely	yellow
c. Friends consult me instead of the weatherman	red

9. Have you had to see a doctor or other health-care provider in the past 3 years for a shoulder problem?

a. No	green
b. One or two visits	yellow
c. I get discount coupons at the orthopaedic office	red

10. Have you ever had a shoulder injury that was severe enough to require a sling and/or keep you out of sports or exercise for an extended period?

a. No	green
b. I was on the shelf, but not for long	yellow
c. I was out of action for a month or more	red

11. Have you ever dislocated or subluxed a shoulder?

a. No	green
b. Yes	red

12. Have you lost mobility (range of motion) in either shoulder? For example, can you fully raise your arm or reach up to scratch your midback?

a. No	green
b. A little stiff at times, but motion is full	yellow
c. Motion is limited in one or more ways	red

13. Have you ever had shoulder surgery?

a. No	green
b. It looms as a possibility	yellow
c. Yes	red

14. Do you awaken at night with your hands or fingers asleep?

a. No	green
b. Rarely, or I easily shake it off	yellow
c. My hand gets more sleep than I do	red

15. Have you had problems with your neck (cervical spine), such as stiffness, tightness, or radiating pain or numbness into the shoulder or arm area?

a. No	green
b. Occasional tightness if I overdo it, but not bad	yellow
c. Neck issues more often than not	red

16. Women, have you ever been pregnant?

a. Never	green
b. Yes, but no problems	yellow
c. Yes, and my body has never been the same	red

17. Women, did you have any significant musculoskeletal problems (such as neck pain, shoulder pain, or sciatica) during or after pregnancy?

a. No or never pregnant	green
b. Yes, but it was fully resolved after delivery	yellow
c. Yes, and it still bothers me	red

18. Do you have diabetes or elevated cholesterol?

a. Neither	green
b. One or both	red

LIFESTYLE

1. Would you say that you're an optimist?

a. Is there any other way to live?	green
b. Still trying to figure that one out	yellow
c. What's the point? Life stinks	red

2. How stressed out are you?

a. Occasional stress, but I seem to handle it well	green
b. I feel overwhelmed at times	yellow
c. Got a Valium?	red

3. For how many hours at a stretch do you sit at a desk?

a. Less than two	green
b. Two to four	yellow
c. More than four	red

4. What type of work have you done most of your life?

a. Not physically demanding	green
b. Occasional overhead lifting or work	yellow
c. Heavy repetitive overhead lifting or work	red

5. Have you ever smoked?

a. No	green
b. Not in the past 10 years	yellow
c. I'm planning to quit	red

6. Find your spot on the body mass index (BMI) chart; are you significantly overweight?

a. Good weight (BMI below 25)	green
b. Mildly overweight (BMI 25–29.9)	yellow
c. Overweight or obese (BMI over 30)	red

7. Do you find it harder to maintain your ideal weight than 5 years ago?

a. No problema	green
b. I've added 5 or 10 pounds in the past 5 years	yellow
c. Call Jenny Craig, or I'll need a whole new wardrobe	red

Body Mass Index Table

	Normal						Overweight					Obese										Extremely Obese														
BMI	19	20	21	22	23	24	25	26	27	28	29	30	31	32	33	34	35	36	37	38	39	40	41	42	43	44	45	46	47	48	49	50	51	52	53	54
Height (inches)														Body Weight (pounds)																						
58	91	96	100	105	110	115	119	124	129	134	138	143	148	153	158	162	167	172	177	181	186	191	196	201	205	210	215	220	224	229	234	239	244	248	253	258
59	94	99	104	109	114	119	124	128	133	138	143	148	153	158	163	168	173	178	183	188	193	198	203	208	212	217	222	227	232	237	242	247	252	257	262	267
60	97	102	107	112	118	123	128	133	138	143	148	153	158	163	168	174	179	184	189	194	199	204	209	215	220	225	230	235	240	245	250	255	261	266	271	276
61	100	106	111	116	122	127	132	137	143	148	153	158	164	169	174	180	185	190	195	201	206	211	217	222	227	232	238	243	248	254	259	264	269	275	280	285
62	104	109	115	120	126	131	136	142	147	153	158	164	169	175	180	186	191	196	202	207	213	218	224	229	235	240	246	251	256	262	267	273	278	284	289	295
63	107	113	118	124	130	135	141	146	152	158	163	169	175	180	186	191	197	203	208	214	220	225	231	237	242	248	254	259	265	270	278	282	287	293	299	304
64	110	116	122	128	134	140	145	151	157	163	169	174	180	186	192	197	204	209	215	221	227	232	238	244	250	256	262	267	273	279	285	291	296	302	308	314
65	114	120	126	132	138	144	150	156	162	168	174	180	186	192	198	204	210	216	222	228	234	240	246	252	258	264	270	276	282	288	294	300	306	312	318	324
66	118	124	130	136	142	148	155	161	167	173	179	186	192	198	204	210	216	223	229	235	241	247	253	260	266	272	278	284	291	297	303	309	315	322	328	334
67	121	127	134	140	146	153	159	166	172	178	185	191	198	204	211	217	223	230	236	242	249	255	261	268	274	280	287	293	299	306	312	319	325	331	338	344
68	125	131	138	144	151	158	164	171	177	184	190	197	203	210	216	223	230	236	243	249	256	262	269	276	282	289	295	302	308	315	322	328	335	341	348	354
69	128	135	142	149	155	162	169	176	182	189	196	203	209	216	223	230	236	243	250	257	263	270	277	284	291	297	304	311	318	324	331	338	345	351	358	365
70	132	139	146	153	160	167	174	181	188	195	202	209	216	222	229	236	243	250	257	264	271	278	285	292	299	306	313	320	327	334	341	348	355	362	369	376
71	136	143	150	157	165	172	179	186	193	200	208	215	222	229	236	243	250	257	265	272	279	286	293	301	308	315	322	329	338	343	351	358	365	372	379	386
72	140	147	154	162	169	177	184	191	199	206	213	221	228	235	242	250	258	265	272	279	287	294	302	309	316	324	331	338	346	353	361	368	375	383	390	397
73	144	151	159	166	174	182	189	197	204	212	219	227	235	242	250	257	265	272	280	288	295	302	310	318	325	333	340	348	355	363	371	378	386	393	401	408
74	148	155	163	171	179	186	194	202	210	218	225	233	241	249	256	264	272	280	287	295	303	311	319	326	334	342	350	358	365	373	381	389	396	404	412	420
75	152	160	168	176	184	192	200	208	216	224	232	240	248	256	264	272	279	287	295	303	311	319	327	335	343	351	359	367	375	383	391	399	407	415	423	431
76	156	164	172	180	189	197	205	213	221	230	238	246	254	263	271	279	287	295	304	312	320	328	336	344	353	361	369	377	385	394	402	410	418	426	435	443

Source: Adapted from *Clinical Guidelines on the Identification, Evaluation, and Treatment of Overweight and Obesity in Adults: The Evidence Report.*

8. Can you pinch an inch around your waist?

a. No	green
b. Yes, when seated	yellow
c. Yes, standing, too	red

9. Do you routinely need to take Advil, Aleve, or Motrin for shoulder discomfort?

a. No	green
b. Once or twice a month	yellow
c. I'm thinking of getting a job at CVS for the discount	red

10. Do you take prescription narcotic drugs for shoulder or neck pain?

a. No	green
b. On rare occasions (i.e., a few times per year)	yellow
c. Pretty regularly, or almost every day and/or for extended periods	red

11. If you're using your arm in a vigorous manner, i.e., throwing, lifting weights, or working, does it fatigue easily or go numb?

a. Never	green
b. Only if I'm pushing	yellow
c. Happens routinely in one or both arms	red

12. How often do you work out?

a. Three times a week, an hour a day	green
b. Maybe once or twice a week	yellow
c. I've been meaning to join a gym	red

13. What does your workout consist of?

a. Balanced routines including aerobic, strengthening, stretching, and core work	green
b. A little of this, a little of that	yellow
c. Mostly one thing (running, swimming, weights)	red

14. Does your upper-body workout include rear deltoid and scapula exercises?

a. Yup, I work on everything	green
b. Not usually	yellow
c. Huh? What's a scapula? I only work on "mirror muscles"	red

15. For a given sport or activity (bicycling, inline skating), do you wear the full protective gear suggested?

a. Yes	green
b. Usually	yellow
c. No	red

16. Do you stop an activity when you feel pain?

a. Always	green
b. Usually	yellow
c. "No pain, no gain" is my mantra	red

17. Are your joints hypermobile? See if you can (without forcing):

Hyperextend your elbows (make them go beyond straight)

Hyperextend your knees (make them go beyond straight)

Pull your thumb all the way backward to touch your forearm or pull your fingers all the way back so they

are at a right angle (or beyond) to your hand

a. My joints do not hyperextend	green
b. One or more joints are loose or slightly hyperextend	yellow
c. Call me Gumby!	red

18. Do you consume more than two glasses of wine (or other alcoholic beverages) a day?

a. Never	green
b. Maybe twice a month	yellow
c. Once or twice a week	red

19. Do you eat breakfast?

a. Religiously	green
b. Sometimes	yellow
c. Who has time?	red

20. Is it a healthful breakfast?

a. With fruit, whole grains, and skim milk or yogurt	green
b. Coffee and toast	yellow
c. None, or coffee and a doughnut or bagel	red

21. What's your daily consumption of fruit and vegetables?

a. Seven to nine servings and a rainbow of colors	green
b. Maybe a green salad with dinner	yellow
c. I don't really like vegetables; do Froot Loops count?	red

22. How often do you eat oily, cold-water fish, such as salmon or sardines?

a. Once or twice a week	green
b. A couple of times a month	yellow
c. There's not much fresh fish where I live	red

23. When you eat on the run, where do you go?

a. Indian, Thai, Japanese, or Greek	green
b. Does the salad bar count?	yellow
c. Would you like fries with that?	red

24. Do you take an antioxidant supplement that includes beta-carotene and vitamins A, C, and E?

a. Daily	green
b. Most of the time	yellow
c. That's just for health nuts from California	red

25. Do you take a multivitamin?

a. Daily	green
b. Most of the time	yellow
c. I thought vitamins were for kids	red

26. Combining food and supplements, do you routinely consume 1,200 milligrams of calcium every day?

a. Yes	green
b. I usually drink some milk and eat some yogurt	yellow
c. I'm not sure	red

27. Do you routinely drink sodas?

a. Never	green
b. Only the diet stuff, and only now and then	yellow
c. I'm a colaholic	red

28. How much water do you take in daily?

a. Eight full glasses	green
b. Four to six glasses, usually	yellow
c. There must be camels in my family tree	red

29. How much sleep do you get each night?

a. 6 to 8 hours	green
b. One hour over or under that span	yellow
c. A lot more (or a lot less)	red

30. Is your sleep restful?

a. I can't wait to face each day	green
b. I often wake up tired, and some afternoons really drag	yellow
c. I check the clock during the night a lot more than I'd like	red

31. Do you snore?

a. Never	green
b. Sometimes	yellow
c. My spouse is ready to toss me out	red

GET PHYSICAL

Caution: These tests may not be easy, but they should be comfortable and not result in any pain. If you feel significant discomfort with any of these tests, or if you are unable to perform one or more of them, *stop* doing those tests and score a "red." Then check with your physician or other health-care professional.

The same rules apply here that apply to any good workout:

■ Warm up before you begin.

■ Slow, controlled movements

SHOULDER THIS

There's an interactive comprehensive self-test for your entire frame, with forms you can print out, on my Web site, www. DrNick.com.

■ No bouncing or ballistic movements

■ No forcing beyond comfort

■ No pain

■ If something doesn't feel right in your shoulder, or anywhere, don't push things.

■ Remember: It's not a competition.

Stork (Basic Balance)

Stand up straight, extend your arms out wide to your sides, then raise one foot off the floor up to the level of the opposite knee (see photo). Rest the arch of your foot on the inner side of your knee, so your legs form the letter P. Now close your eyes. Repeat on the opposite side. How long can you stay balanced with eyes closed?

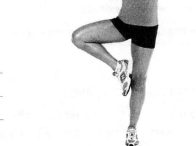

a. 30 seconds	green
b. 15–30 seconds	yellow
c. Less than 15 seconds	red

Forearm Flexibility

Extend your arms directly in front of you, elbows straight and hands up like a traffic officer saying "stop." Your hands should be perfectly vertical, your wrists making a 90-degree angle without any discomfort or strain. Now try the same thing palms down. Again, your wrists should be able to make a 90-degree angle. Can you make a 90-degree angle?

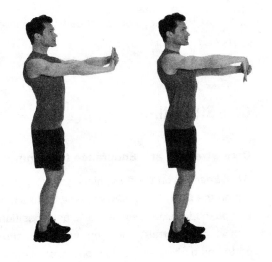

a. Yes	green
b. No	red

Neck Rotation (Cervical Spine)

Stand sideways to a mirror and look at yourself over your shoulder. Can you turn a full 90 degrees so that your nose is in line with your shoulder (on *both* sides)?

a. Yes	green
b. Very, very close	yellow
c. No	red

Neck Flexion (Cervical Spine)

Look straight ahead; now slowly look downward and try to touch your chin to your breastbone. Can you do it?

a. Chin touches breastbone easily	green
b. Chin is one finger-width away from breastbone	yellow
c. No way	red

Neck Extension (Cervical Spine)

Looking in the mirror, touch your forefinger to the tip of your nose and hold it in that exact spot. Then tilt your head back slowly, looking toward the ceiling, to see if you can get your entire chin above the level of your fingertip. Do not lean back; only your head should be moving. Can you do it?

a. Yes	green
b. Almost there (i.e., chin reaches fingertip level)	yellow
c. No way	red

Core Strength

Core Strength and Endurance (Quadruped)

While kneeling on the floor, place your forearms flat on the floor as if you were going to do a modified pushup. Next, assume the "plank" position with your body straight and your full weight supported on both forearms and toes (first photo). Your body should be straight as a board, your pelvis tucked inward, tightening your abdominal and buttock muscles. Try holding this position with your weight on your forearms and toes for 60 seconds.

Next, lift your right arm off the floor for 15 seconds, supporting your full weight on your left arm and both feet (second photo). Repeat, lifting your left arm.

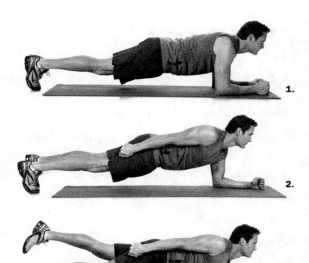

1.

2.

3.

With both forearms on the floor, raise your right leg, hold for 15 seconds, and then repeat, lifting your left leg (not shown).

Next, try to elevate your right arm and left leg simultaneously (third photo) and hold for 15 seconds, then return them to the floor and repeat with your left arm and right leg raised. Return to the plank position and hold for another 30 seconds.

How did it go?

a. Able to do all positions for the required time	green
b. Able to do all positions for half of the required time	yellow
c. Unable to hold all or any positions other than briefly	red

Side Plank

Start on the floor lying on your left side, propping yourself up on your left forearm with your left elbow in line with your left shoulder, and your left outer thigh and leg on the floor with your feet lying stacked, one on the other. Your right arm should rest over your right hip. Press your hips toward the ceiling and lift your body off the floor so as to form a straight line while balancing on your forearm and the side of your foot. Hold this position while contracting your abdominals to stabilize your torso. Breathe comfortably and don't hold your breath. Try to tighten your abs and gluteal (butt) muscles simultaneously, but keep your shoulders relaxed. Time yourself as you hold this position for as long as you can comfortably, without sagging or squirming. Now try this on the opposite side. How long could you hold it?

a. 3 minutes	green
b. Less than 2 minutes	yellow
c. Less than 30 seconds or can't do	red

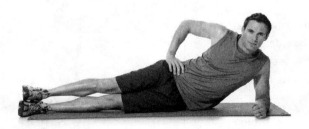 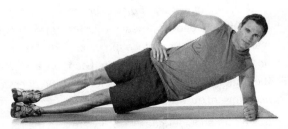

Shoulder Reach

Reach behind your back, with one hand coming from above, over your shoulder, and the other hand reaching up from behind the small of your back. Now reverse arm positions and try again. What can you do on *both* sides?

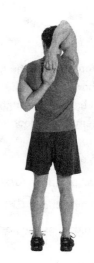

a. Clasp my hands	green
b. Touch my fingertips	yellow
c. Are you joking?	red

Statue of Liberty

Lie on your back on the floor, with your arms relaxed at your sides. Raise one arm up and over your head with the elbow straight until it comes back down in a full arc toward the floor, as if you're doing the backstroke, only with your palm up toward the ceiling in the "Statue of Liberty" position. Repeat with the other arm. What can you do?

a. Shoulder, elbow, and wrist all touch floor	green
b. Wrist is 2 inches or less off the floor	yellow
c. Wrist "hangs up" more than 2 inches off the floor	red

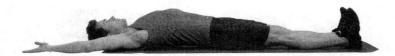

Doorjamb Stretch

Caution: Do not perform this test if you have significant shoulder instability with history of dislocations.

Stand in a doorway. Reach your arm up so that the elbow is at shoulder height. Now place the inner part of your elbow, forearm, and open palm on the doorjamb. Lean forward, feeling a stretch on the front of your shoulder. How far past the door does your shoulder bend inward/forward?

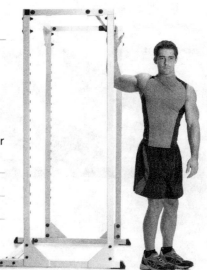

a. Front of shoulder goes well forward into the room	green
b. Front of shoulder just about reaches doorway level	yellow
c. Front of shoulder hardly moves forward	red

Sleeper Stretch

Lie on the floor or on a bed on your left side, with your left arm pointing straight out in front of you (at the same level as the shoulder), with the elbow bent 90 degrees and your hand pointing upward. Using your right hand, gently push your left hand downward toward the floor or bed (while your shoulder rotates). See how far you can go without forcing things. Switch sides and try the other arm.

a. Open palm goes easily to the floor or bed	green
b. Open palm almost hits the floor or bed (i.e., 1 or 2 inches away)	yellow
c. Arm hangs up and palm is far from the floor or bed	red

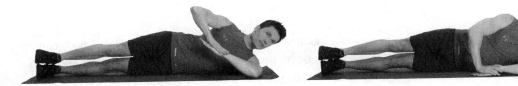

Side Raise

Stand with your arms at your sides. Slowly raise your straightened left arm out to your side. Continue to raise it, like the second hand going around on a clock, until your fingers are pointing up at the ceiling. Next, lower your arm and try with your right side. As you raise your arm, especially when your hand reaches shoulder height, how do you feel?

a. Fine, smooth ride	green
b. Catches a little midway, but better as it goes all the way up	yellow
c. Pain and difficulty—something not right in there	red

Upper-Body Strength—*Pushups*

Men should do the standard "military-style" pushup, with only the hands and toes (not knees) touching the floor. Women have the additional option of using the kneeling or "bent-knee" position (kneel on the floor, hands forward on the floor, keeping your back straight). Do as many pushups as possible without stopping, until you can no longer do any with good form. Keep your back straight and let your chest touch the floor on the way down—no bouncing. Count the total number of pushups performed.

	MEN	WOMEN	
a.	>25	>18	green
b.	12–25	7–18	yellow
c.	<12	<7	red

Shoulder Posture

Stand the way you *normally* do (that is, don't cheat!), sideways to a mirror with your shirt off. Check for shoulder position (i.e., is your shoulder hunched forward?) and front-to-back muscle symmetry.

a. My shoulder is pretty centered, and the muscles in the back (rear deltoid) are as full as the ones in the front	green
b. My shoulders are a little forward, and the muscles look pretty equal in the front and back	yellow
c. My shoulders are hunched quite forward, and most of the muscle mass is in the front	red

Body Posture

The final item on your self-test is an overall evaluation of how you carry your body—or your body carries you—and how you present yourself to the world. Get down to some tights or your underwear and have your partner snap a picture of you from the side while you stand as you naturally would (it's best if the photo is taken when you least expect it). Then place a ruler over the photo and draw a line from the back of your ear to your heel. Ideally, the line should bisect your shoulder, pass through your hip, and graze the back of your leg at the knee. How does your image look?

a. Straight as a soldier	green
b. A little stooped	yellow
c. Gee, I didn't think I resembled the Hunchback of Notre Dame	red

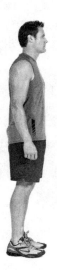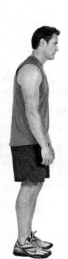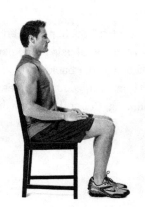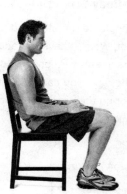

Now, have a photo taken—again, when least expected—while you're sitting naturally on a straight-backed, armless chair. This photo could best be described as:

a. The epitome of good posture	green
b. A bit bent over, but that usually is only when I'm tired	yellow
c. Call me slouch	red

Totals   **Green:** _____   **Yellow:** _____   **Red:** _____

ASSESSMENT

Similar to the self-tests in other FrameWork publications and the FrameWork *Active for Life* book series, the above self-evaluation is not so much about a particular "score": It's about identifying and focusing on critical areas that need your attention so you can lead a more active life. It's less about whether you have passed or failed, and more about raising your awareness about the many things that contribute to having a healthy frame.

The more reds you have, the more serious shoulder-related risk you have. If you didn't circle any reds but you have a passel of yellows, you're at high risk of slipping into one or more red classifications in the not-too-distant future. If you had just a couple of yellows and the rest were green, you're in good shape, and it won't take much effort to get into top shape. If you circled nothing but green, give yourself a pat on the back (shouldn't be hard for you to do that, given your great shoulder mobility). You should count on progressing rapidly into the more advanced shoulder program.

What's most important to take away from this exercise is that regardless of what shape you're in, it can be better. Any frame can be made stronger, and any weak links can be "toughened," modified, or at least managed better—albeit some more easily than others. (You can monitor your progress by repeating this self-test regularly and paying special attention to those questions you answered with a yellow or red.) Take the next two steps and you will extend your warranty and make yourself far less vulnerable down the road, able to rely on the frame you were born with a whole lot longer.

SHOULDER SHOULDS

I always look forward to this step because it's an opportunity to point out once again the core of the FrameWork philosophy: *prevention*. And that gives me another opportunity to repeat several of those doctor recommendations that never go out of style.

The shoulder exercises in the next chapter are a fantastic prescription for keeping another frame part in tip-top shape, but being active for life requires a lot more than a targeted workout. It requires a healthy lifestyle, balanced training, core fitness, proper rest and recovery, and a sound mind. In other words, it requires a foundation that supports general health over the long haul. That weekly golf or tennis date or regular visits to the local gym won't extend your frame's warranty the way the comprehensive approach herein does.

There are no shortcuts if you want to enjoy the best of health. You must address all of the aspects above that affect well-being, and when you take this step, you will have done all you can to avoid illness and injury: You will have given yourself every chance to be active for life. Even if you're a FrameWork veteran, it's always a good idea to revisit the absolutes of frame health. At the top of that list is the subject of widespread public-service messages.

SMOKE GETS IN YOUR BONES

Doctors and health officials won't stop beating the antismoking drum until the nastiest of habits is a thing of the past for everyone. It bears repeating here that blood-vessel constriction caused by smoke inhalation has been linked to poor bone healing and a variety of other negative musculoskeletal consequences, and that many orthopaedic surgeons now say they won't operate on someone unless he or she quits.

Smokers have poor bone healing because

bones have to rely on microcirculation, a network of tiny capillaries that is constricted by smoke. Smoking slows or prevents bone healing (what we doctors refer to as delayed unions, or nonunions), and smokers have a higher incidence of shoulder rotator cuff injuries (yes, smoke gets in your shoulders as well!), degenerative disks, and other frame problems. Even passive smoke exposure could instantly shut down the microvascular network of blood vessels. So quit *now*, and shun all who partake. You'll be doing yourself, and them, a favor.

HEAVY BREATHING

Any program to improve health must include moderate aerobic exercise for 30 minutes at least three times per week, and your shoulder program is no exception. When your blood is pumping, it finds its way into the nooks and

Off the Cuff

When I was a resident in training, hand surgeons were just starting to reattach severed fingers with microvascular surgery, known as replanting. That was the era when you actually could smoke in hospitals— and we'd notice that if somebody was smoking a cigarette as he or she walked by the room of a patient who had had a replant, the reattached finger turned blue!

Motion is lotion.

crannies deep in the shoulder, lubricating and warming things up—something critical for those with shoulder ailments and anyone over 40. In general, your heart can't tell the difference between different aerobic activities (they all help improve cardiac health and function), but your frame can, because it will certainly have its preferences depending on what ails you. Running is great, but it delivers a pounding to your aging frame. Those with lower-body musculoskeletal ailments like hip or knee arthritis should pay special attention to this fact; everyone should know that there are other options to get your blood moving that are a lot easier on your entire frame:

Walking

Wear comfortable shoes with good support and cushion—I prefer running sneakers to those designed for walking—and start at a slow pace for 5 minutes to warm up. Increase to a medium pace for 10 minutes, and gradually build up to 30 minutes by adding a few minutes each day. Cool down with 5 minutes at a slow pace. After a few weeks, increase intensity by increasing the pace and/or swinging your arms as you walk. (If it's difficult to talk while you walk, you may be overextending yourself—dial it back a notch.)

Water Workouts

If you have access to a pool, swimming, walking or jogging in the water, and water-aerobic routines are terrific low-impact exercise options, especially for those who are overweight or have shoulder woes. For a more intense workout, add weights to the ankles or flipper-type paddles to the hands. (Freestyle swimming can be problematic for those with rotator cuff problems, so your water workouts may need some adjustment until things improve or resolve in the shoulder area.)

Stationary Bike

Your seat should be high enough so that your knees are almost but not fully locked out when the pedal is at its lowest. (A recumbent bike is used in a reclining position that some find more comfortable.)

Elliptical Trainer

This machine is a cross between a stationary bike and a stairclimber, and when the arms

are also used (i.e., not just resting on the handles), it provides a higher-intensity cardio workout, as it works all of the frame's primary muscle groups. It also brings more immediate bloodflow to the upper body and shoulder.

If the activities above aren't your cup of tea, take a bicycle to and from work or local stores, or just take it for a long ride around your neighborhood. Try jumping rope or jumping jacks (terrific shoulder "warmers"). If your knees aren't an issue, by all means enjoy jogging or more intense running. No matter how you do it, get your heart pumping and your frame primed for the other exercise it needs.

BALANCED TRAINING

"Mirror muscles" might look terrific, but they're not as beautiful as they could be if lesser muscles and the cardiovascular system aren't given a regular workout. In fact, mirror muscles might actually work against you if they are overdeveloped, because they can cause weaker, neglected areas to "pop" more than they would if all soft tissue were properly balanced. This is especially true in the shoulder, where front-to-back strength imbalances are extremely commonplace, particularly in guys doing lots of strength training. (No wonder there are so many shoulder problems in the "iron warriors"!) It is just as important to work on strengthening rear deltoid, rear cuff, and scapular (shoulder blade) areas as well as stretching the *front* of the shoulder.

Running and other strenuous aerobic activities can also create imbalances. For example, a lot of runners only like to run and will typically have great hearts and very strong calves, but they usually have extremely tight hamstrings, a tight lower back, tight front shoulders, and relatively weak abdominals—so they're set up for back, hip, and shoulder problems. Their frames are out of balance because of the disparities created by the repetitive act of running.

If you're a gym rat or a runner, that's great—I'd be the last one to stop anyone from working out. For comprehensive frame health, however, you have to do some cross-training that includes targeted stretching, core exercises, and strengthening of all muscle groups to stay out of trouble with any frame part. (For more in-depth information about balanced training and comprehensive fitness, please see Additional Resources on page 195.)

ACTIVE R & R

Fierce dedication to exercise is laudable, but proper recovery from exercise is a step that is often overlooked by many health-minded individuals. And if you're one of those who think that just alternating workout activities—aerobic training one day, anaerobic the next—is adequate for recovery, you've got another think coming, because at times your entire body needs to be shut down.

As you go on, you aren't aware that overall stress accumulates in your body. Exercises might be directed at one area, but there is a

SHOULDER THIS

Lao-Tzu on Overexertion
(from the *Tao Te Ching*)
A bow that is stretched
to its fullest capacity
may certainly snap.
A sword that is tempered
to its very sharpest
may easily be broken.

cumulative toll on your system that can cause an overall crash or one of the overuse injuries we talked about earlier. Overtraining syndrome and overuse injuries are preventable if you give your body the rest that it needs after life-giving—but strenuous—exercise.

Rest must occur both locally (i.e., the muscles that were worked) and systemically (from an overall metabolic standpoint). Exercise is a powerful stimulus that creates spectacular changes in your body and frame, but those positive changes occur during the rest and recovery period, a critical time for making gains. Come back too soon and apply another stimulus before adequate recovery occurs, and you're asking for a breakdown. It's a lot like cell phones and PDAs—they've transformed how we live and how we communicate, but if you don't routinely recharge the battery, they're useless. This applies to you, too. Take time, and measures, to recharge.

This doesn't mean you should plop into a recliner and put your feet up. There are better ways to recover from exercise:

- Casual walking

- Stretching

- Yoga or tai chi

- Meditation

In other words, you can still *do* something (that's why we call it *active* R & R) to gain the benefit of doing nothing, which can even (sometimes) include plopping on that recliner.

Your nutritional choices (covered in depth in the next section) are also very important in terms of recovery, especially after a hard workout or a few hours of your favorite sport. Muscle recovery is aided by taking in food, drink, or a supplement that contains the right mix of proteins and carbs within 30 minutes of stopping the activity. Interestingly, low-fat chocolate milk has been shown to be a perfect option that aids and optimizes recovery immediately after a hard workout. You should also refuel your muscles later that day with a high-quality, high-carb meal.

Next, the importance of hydration cannot be overstated. It plays a critical role in helping your frame bounce back from the natural wear and tear that exercise causes. Water intake all day long and before, during, and after you exercise is a must, because it oils your body's repair mechanisms and "juices" the synovial fluid in your shoulders.

Last, but not least, proper sleep is critical for recovery. Studies show that those who sleep less than 6 hours, or more than 9, have impaired mental function, are more susceptible to disease, and have higher obesity and even mortality rates. Prolonged periods of disturbed sleep require the attention of a physician. If you are not among the 40 million

SHOULDER THIS

Temporary Sleep Supplements

5-hydroxytryptophan, or 5-HTP (50 mg)

Melatonin (3 mg)

Calcium (300 mg)

Magnesium (500 mg)

Valerian (400 mg)

SHOULDER THIS

Sweet Dreams

■ No caffeine after lunch, and no major meal within 2 hours of bedtime.

■ Leave your work at work!

■ Invest in a good, comfortable mattress.

■ Read just before bedtime—no TV.

who have a chronic sleep disorder, but you have an occasional bout of sleep disturbance (including snoring, a sign of low-quality sleep), light exercise an hour before bedtime is a natural soporific (sleep remedy), and there are some supplements you can take on a temporary basis to get you through (see "Temporary Sleep Supplements").

The lowdown on your shoulder fitness program is the same as that for any other exercise program: Gains in strength, flexibility, durability, and balance happen in your downtime. So take a day, or even two, off, but stay active in other ways and make proper nutrition and sleep a priority.

ACTIVE EATING

For every pound you carry, your body thinks it's 5 (or more, depending on the type of activity) because of compound load stresses, so if you're 10 pounds overweight, it feels like 50 on your frame! Small amounts of extra weight are amplified across your knees, hips, and ankles. Excess pounds on your frame cause and accelerate damage and hamper recovery from injury. They strain connective tissue, grind joints, and play a role in arthritis and other inflammation throughout your body. It isn't a surprise that obesity is also related to certain shoulder disorders, including rotator cuff ailments.

The good news about poundage is that it works both ways—if you lose 5 pounds, your frame thinks you lost 25. That's a pretty good deal when you think about it, and it is why even small amounts of weight loss have been shown to lessen the progression of arthritis.

But losing weight is one thing; keeping it off is quite another, and that's the primary drawback of otherwise excellent diet programs. They simply do not emphasize enough the critical ingredient in any diet: exercise. It's not that the value of exercise isn't known, it's that it's the elephant in the room that few want to talk about. We're all too busy in our daily lives and too sedentary as a rule in our leisure time (albeit with the best intentions to work out regularly "someday"), and wrestling with a diet is often plenty on our "plate."

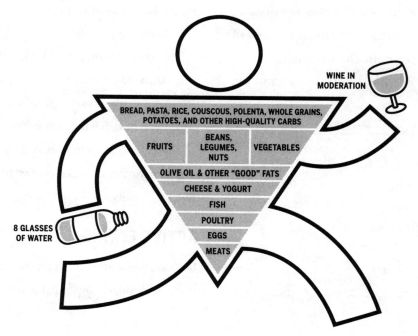

WINE IN MODERATION

BREAD, PASTA, RICE, COUSCOUS, POLENTA, WHOLE GRAINS, POTATOES, AND OTHER HIGH-QUALITY CARBS

FRUITS | BEANS, LEGUMES, NUTS | VEGETABLES

OLIVE OIL & OTHER "GOOD" FATS

CHEESE & YOGURT

FISH

POULTRY

EGGS

MEATS

8 GLASSES OF WATER

Whether or not you're overweight, I'm here to tell you that "someday" must be today because of the way your metabolism works. It was programmed way back in our evolution as a survival mechanism. If you diet and significantly cut back on calories consumed, the body senses starvation and plays a nasty trick on you: It starts to cannibalize muscle first, not fat. Muscles use a lot of calories, so loss of muscle mass lowers your metabolic rate. That makes you hungry, and you're more vulnerable to gaining weight because of the lower metabolic rate (your internal furnace thermostat set point) that you have after you lose muscle.

How can you short-circuit this vicious cycle? With muscle building and toning, which I've found isn't stressed enough in weight-loss discussions and programs.

Complicating these weighty matters is the fact that you will gradually lose muscle and weaken your frame as you age. We're prone to gain weight as we get older because, again, our bodies compensate for muscle loss with hunger pangs. So everyone—no matter how heavy or how old—has to exercise, and their program must include some sort of resistance training to build and/or maintain total body musculature. Such

SHOULDER THIS

Calorie Burn per Hour

Housework—160
Walking—280
Gardening—350
Singles tennis—550
Doubles tennis—350
Aerobics—450
Light jogging—500
Swimming—500
Water polo—700
Hiking—500
Power walking—600
Squash—650
Running—700

training maintains and builds bones and tendons in addition to muscle, and that's what helps keep any excess weight off the frame. With every bit of muscle you add, you raise your metabolic rate and burn more calories, even if you're just sitting around doing nothing.

As for a weight-loss diet, the primary factor is calorie control. Science tells us that a pound is equivalent to 3,500 calories, so if your goal is to lose a pound a week, calorie intake must be reduced by 500 calories each day. This is easier than you would think if you learn to say no to sweet drinks and processed or sweet snacks. Learning to read food labels is critical (see "Off the Cuff" for specifics), and perhaps the most important thing you can do in the battle of the bulge.

Most rapid-weight-loss programs deprive the body of important nutrients, and the "rapid" weight that is lost is usually water and muscle. Not good! The goal is to lose fat and get leaner. Don't look at the scale—look at yourself in the mirror. As a famous body-builder once told me, "If you can't flex it, lose it." I don't think you have to go that far, but you get the message.

Now that you know about the relationship

Off the Cuff

Let's "chew" on food labels for a moment, because they provide a wealth of vital information in addition to calorie counts. Pay careful attention to the facts that calories are *per serving,* and that the package contains a specific number of servings that is listed right at the top of the label. So if you eat a bag of peanuts that contains three servings, and there are 100 calories per serving, you just consumed 300 calories—not 100.

Next, the total-fat category is subdivided into saturated fat and trans fats (what's left after you subtract those two from total fat is usually the fat that is good for you). Stay completely away from trans fats and save saturated fat for a rare, special treat, such as an occasional pat of butter.

Most people should stay under 300 milligrams of cholesterol, the next label category; if you have heart issues or you were told your cholesterol is high, keep it below 200 milligrams per day. Moving down the label, the US recommended dietary allowance (RDA) for sodium is 2,400 milligrams, but research is pushing that number lower, toward the UK's 1,600-milligrams RDA. The RDA for potassium is 3,500 milligrams (a banana has about 400 milligrams; a cup of lima beans is close to 1,000 milligrams).

The all-important total-carbohydrate category, subdivided into dietary fiber and sugars, is next. Very few among us get the 25 grams of fiber per day that is optimum for weight and blood glucose control, so home in on that number when you weigh options on the shelf. Official US guidelines advise a maximum of 40 grams of refined sugar per 2,000 calories, but try to cut that in half. (And note that "refined sugar" isn't just table sugar; it is also the kind that is in a wide range of processed foods such as certain breakfast cereals.)

of calories to pounds, it's a matter of calculating exactly what you consume over a week, and that's not all that tough to do when we consider the almost-universal labeling we have now. So keep a running tab (i.e., a food diary) of *everything* you put into your mouth over 7 days, without changing your usual eating routine. (Pay particular attention to your choice of beverages. Stick with water most of the time and cut out any sweet drinks, which are loaded with "naked" calories.)

Whatever your weekly consumption number turns out to be, divide it by 7, subtract 500, and that's your daily allotment that guarantees you'll lose weight. (I'll let you in on a little secret: Your 500-calorie

---

Last but not least are the protein and vitamin categories. The RDA for protein is 0.8 grams per kilogram (2.2 pounds) of body weight, and that is between 40 grams and 70 grams per day for most people. If you're pregnant or in the older crowd, you'll need a little more (consult your physician), and a 50 percent increase in your recommended daily protein intake is recommended if you train hard. Most of us don't get enough protein in our daily diets. Look for high-quality protein sources, and even supplement with a shake if needed. As for vitamins? Get as many and as much of them as you can.

The labels will also say whether food items have peanuts, lactose, or other products that can cause severe allergic reactions. (My daughter Emily is allergic to peanuts, so she learned as a youngster to scan the labels of any foods she wasn't familiar with, and this has helped her become a nutrition guru at a very young age. She often has me put back certain things as she reminds me of what's on the label. Thank you, Emily!)

Proper nutrition is not so much about any one thing you eat as it is about getting used to what labels tell you and thinking about what you are putting into your body each day. For example, if you like pretzels, most brands are okay, but some have a ton of salt and/or bad fats to tantalize the tastebuds. Whatever product you are buying, compare labels side by side and choose wisely. If labels are a case of TMI for you, some nutritionists will gladly go on a field trip to the local supermarket with you to give you a "healthy" course on how to use them. That's what sports nutritionist Jeanie Subach does routinely for some players on the Philadelphia Eagles, Philadelphia Flyers, and Philadelphia 76ers. If they can do it, so can you.

reduction doesn't have to come solely from giving up some food. Exercise of any kind burns calories in varying degrees; 20 minutes of walking makes about 80 calories disappear, 20 minutes of vigorous gardening lops off 100 plus, and the same time spent doing strenuous aerobics burns 150 or more. That's a good thing, because if you're like me, you cherish every bite you take and might have a very tough time doing without some favorites.)

There really isn't any magic involved in slimming down. It has nothing to do with a narrow focus on low carbs, all protein, good fats, or the new fad diet that either starves you or bores you to tears. It's about watching what you eat and taking advantage of the excellent nutrition in all food groups. I recommend the Mediterranean diet because it has everything you need and never bores the tastebuds or the stomach, and it's great for your frame with all its natural antioxidant and anti-inflammatory ingredients. There are other diets that are balanced, with good carbs, friendly fats, and anti-inflammatory foods, so eat whatever you like—up to your limit and in proportion with the FrameWork Pyramid that maximizes grains and minimizes meat and eggs.

YOUR FRAMEWORK TRAINING TABLE

If you are what you just ate, you will be what you eat from now on. Again, you can choose what you eat, but you must choose wisely; you must include in your diet every major food group and every color of the rainbow. I'll leave the specifics about a menu up to you, but I've got some general guidelines that will help you to maximize nutritional value:

■ A good rule of thumb is to allocate 20 percent of your diet to protein, 15 percent to polyunsaturated fats, 10 percent to monounsaturated fats, and 55 percent to good carbs. When you make your choices from the latter category, give the nod every time to the ones highest in fiber content, because you should be consuming 25 grams of fiber each day.

■ Muscles require amino acids, those protein building blocks, and our protein needs increase with age because of the associated muscle loss. Protein is always necessary to replenish muscle fibers, yet protein is not as well absorbed into your system as you get older. The fact is, young or old, most of us do not take in enough protein. Why? Because we've all been cutting way back on red meat and eggs to reduce the risk of cardiovascular disease, and we haven't substituted enough of the better protein choices

SHOULDER THIS

GOOD CARBS

Whole grain bread, cereal, pasta

Brown rice, couscous, chickpeas, lentils

Oat bran

Leafy vegetables

Seeds (pumpkin, sesame, sunflower, flax)

Fruit (especially pineapple, grapefruit, cherries, unsweetened strawberries, peaches, and cantaloupe)

SHOULDER THIS

Friendly Fats

POLYUNSATURATED

Safflower, sunflower, corn, soybean oils

Walnuts

Oily fish

MONOUNSATURATED

Extra-virgin olive oil, canola oil

Avocados

Peanuts, hazelnuts, almonds, cashews

to make up the difference. Look for lean protein: chicken and turkey without the skin and salt (and hold the mayo, too), wild salmon, trout, herring, anchovies and sardines, or soy if you're a vegetarian. Mix in more brown rice, beans, and lentils to make up any protein shortfall.

■ We've all been warned about the dangers associated with butter, cheese, cream, and whole milk, but make sure some of your menu choices include good fats. The medical literature is peppered with studies that confirm the efficacy of the omega-3 fatty acids in olive oil, oily fish, nuts, and seeds—staples of the Mediterranean diet. They're a boon to cardiovascular health, but they come with an advisory: Fats are extremely high in calories—200 in only ¼ cup of some nuts, for example—so measure quantities very carefully. The upside is that a small amount goes a long way toward curbing your appetite. (As an appetizer or snack, try a couple of tablespoons of hummus with half of a whole wheat pita, or a sliced banana with some flaxseed sprinkled on it, and see for yourself.)

■ Good diets eliminate the carbs that aren't good for us—fried potatoes, white bread, white rice, sugar—but the best diet is loaded with carbs that fuel your frame while they fill your stomach—whole grains, leafy vegetables, fruit, and seeds. You don't have to totally give up bread and pasta, just make them a special treat, and, yes, you can indulge in the nutrition-rich potato— preferably boiled, steamed, or baked. Remember: The main fuel of choice for Olympic athletes is carbs. It really makes no sense to me when individuals who want to get fit, and look better, cut out carbs completely. For them I have two words: Michael Phelps. When training, this young hero consumes more than 12,000 carb-loaded calories a day!

SHOULDER THIS

The Rainbow of Nutrition

RED: Tomatoes, red peppers, pink grapefruit, watermelon

REDDISH ORANGE: Carrots, mangoes, cantaloupe, winter squash, sweet potatoes

YELLOW/ORANGE: Peaches, papaya, nectarines, pineapple

YELLOW/GREEN: Spinach, corn, green peas, avocado, honeydew melon

GREEN: Broccoli, brussels sprouts, cabbage, kale, bok choy

WHITE/GREEN: Garlic, onions, leeks, celery, asparagus, pears, green grapes

PURPLE: Blueberries, plums, beets, eggplant, red cabbage

■ Next on the FrameWork menu are foods that minimize inflammation and oxidation. It's no coincidence that the protein, good carbs, and friendly fats discussed above provide not only the right, balanced nutrition, but also decrease inflammatory and cell-destructive reactions in your body. It is no wonder that the Mediterranean diet is recommended for individuals with arthritis, for instance, because it is packed with anti-inflammatory nutrients. (You might have noticed that junk food, fried food, saturated and partially hydrogenated fats, baked goods, and sweets are nowhere to be found in the diet recommendations here. Those food selections should be avoided like the plague because of the systemic havoc they wreak in your body. They promote the enemy, inflammation, which can be destructive to both your heart and your frame parts.)

■ Accent your menu with a wide variety of spices that don't add calories to your plate and make your food tastier as they deliver antioxidation and anti-inflammation support.

■ Last but not least, a word about hydration. Water makes digestion possible; it is a solvent for nutrients and transports them everywhere. It assists muscle contraction and serves as a shock absorber all over your body, especially in those disks between vertebrae. Water regulates your body temperature and eliminates waste products. And, for all you weight battlers out there, it fills you up and neutralizes food cravings.

Your blood is 90 percent water, your brain is 85 percent water, your muscles are 72 percent water, and your skin is 71 percent water. A water deficiency shows up as

reduced mental acuity, fatigue, wrinkled skin, or the muscle cramps that both professional athletes and regular folks sometimes get when engaging in sports. If you feel plumb tuckered out, have a headache or eye strain, or have sore muscles in your neck and back, it might have nothing at all to do with overwork and stress—it just might be a serious lack of aqua.

Bottom line? You need to drink 2 quarts of water every day. As it is with fiber, however, many among us don't consume as much as we should. So be like those people you see all around who have a water bottle in their hand, cup holder, or carry-all or on their desk. (Drinks that contain caffeine don't count—caffeine is a diuretic that drains body fluid. If you've had your fill of water, try grape, cherry, açai, goji, or pomegranate juice; teas that don't contain caffeine; or smoothies made in a blender with fruit, ice, and low-fat yogurt.)

Supplemental Nutritional Advice

Even if you always eat only the best things, your gastrointestinal system is inefficient—it can't extract all the good nutrients from the food you ingest. This, coupled with taste preferences that may inadvertently be causing you to miss out on something your frame needs, is why every diet must include some basic over-the-counter (OTC) supplements.

But beware, you bargain shoppers out there—supplements, unlike pharmaceutical-grade drugs, do not have to meet label claims. Many companies use foreign suppliers whose ingredients have less-than-advertised potency, and some use additional substances not on the label that could be quite harmful to you, especially if you are taking any prescription medication. The brand matters—buy only from reputable manufacturers that conform to strict codes regarding product quality and labeling. The best companies earn the United States Pharmacopeia (USP) seal of approval. Also, competitive athletes, beware: Hidden substances or impurities can result in a drug-test violation and a stripped medal or victory. Look for supplements that are "Certified for Sport," like Cosamin DS and Cosamin ASU from Nutramax Labs. These joint supplements can be very useful in the shoulder, where arthritis seems to be more and more common. I even have some patients with rotator cuff issues (whom I placed on joint supplements for knee arthritis) who tell me that their shoulder tendon problems have improved. Perhaps it is the anti-inflammatory properties of these natural substances, especially those with ASU (avocado-soybean unsaponifiable), that deliver benefit.

In addition to a broad-spectrum multivitamin, a program that buttresses your diet and bolsters your frame covers three vital areas: bone/connective tissue support, inflammation control, and antioxidant protection. (Check "Supplement Your Frame" for specifics.)

Digestive inefficiencies also explain in part those hunger pangs we get now and then. One diet trick you can stick to is splitting your daily protein allowance over two or three meals; protein takes longer to break down, so you feel full longer. Another trick is to allocate 20 to 40 percent of your daily calorie allowance to healthy snacks. Many people find that having multiple smaller meals spread throughout the day keeps them satisfied and lessens the urge to binge at regular mealtimes. This approach also tends to keep blood sugar and insulin levels more stable throughout the day. Get in the habit of having a baggie with some goodies (seeds, raisins, celery, carrots, broccoli, grapes) handy so you don't end up with a soda or candy bar to satisfy a craving with 300 or more of those empty calories.

Yes, weight management and healthy nutrition come down to the choices you make every day about what you will put into your mouth—both quantity and quality. You'll either increase your fat, your blood sugar, your weight, and inflammatory reactions in your

SHOULDER THIS

Supplement Your Frame

BONE/CONNECTIVE TISSUE SUPPORT

Glucosamine/chondroitin (1,500 mg/1,200 mg)*

Calcium (1,200 mg)

Vitamin D_3 (1,000 IU)

L-arginine (1,600 mg)

L-glutamine (1,000 mg)

Avocado-soybean unsaponifiable (300 mg)*

MSM (3,000 mg)

ANTIOXIDANT PROTECTION

Pycnogenol (pine bark extract, 100 mg)

CoQ_{10} (50 mg)

Grapeseed extract (100mg) with resveratrol (20 mg)

L-glutathione (reduced form, 100 mg)

Green tea

INFLAMMATION CONTROL

Avocado-soybean unsaponifiable (300 mg)*

Curcumin (400 mg)

Quercetin (500 mg)

S-adenosylmethionine (SAM-e, 800 mg)

Willow bark (1,600 mg)

Gamma linolenic acid (GLA, 250 mg)

Flaxseed (2,000 mg)

Resveratrol** (also in red grapes and red wine)

*I recommend the Cosamin DS and Cosamin ASU formulations from Nutramax Labs (www.nutramaxlabs.com).

**I recommend Bioforte from Biotivia (www.biotivia.com).

muscles and joints, or reduce them with the help of Mother Nature. Acquire better food habits and make better choices: extra-virgin oil and vinegar instead of Caesar salad dressing; teas and unsweetened juices instead of soda that blocks calcium absorption because of its phosphorus content; dark honey or stevia instead of sugar; mustard instead of mayo; spices instead of salt; fresh food prepared fast instead of fast food. (And don't forget to grab a cup of water every chance you get.)

Eat well and have fun doing it. It's a great way to extend your frame's warranty.

MIND MATTERS

Sports-medicine doctors know that psychological issues are important in dealing with orthopaedic problems and injuries, and yet history has shown that many if not most of us aren't very good at doing anything about them. There are times when I walk into an examination room, and before I even know what the patient's issue is, I have a feeling, a sixth sense, that I won't be able to help. I know that the right diagnosis and treatment won't be enough to get that person better because there are emotional or other psychosocial issues involved. That "baggage" hasn't been checked.

Orthopaedic specialists are aware of the importance of a patient's mind "frame." We've seen the same studies every other doctor has that unequivocally connect stress with immune dysfunction, disease, and pain tolerance, even changes in brain function and brain-wave activity, but we haven't connected all the dots on how to help patients who are stressed out. Mind and body tend to be seen as two completely different and completely separate realms. We, as surgeons, all too often just deal with the physical; we don't get patients to the right person, or incorporate a team approach, or, perhaps most important of all, call on them to help themselves emotionally. The result is suboptimal healing and/or recovery and recurrent frame-related (or other) ailments.

That's beginning to change in a big way. Psychoneuroimmunology (PNI) is a medical discipline, still in its formative stages, that was established to clarify the complex hormonal and biochemical triggers that alter the immune response and other physiological systems. These triggers either allow your mind and central nervous system to give you a boost or set off a downward spiral.

Helen Flanders Dunbar, MD, said, "It's not a question of whether an illness is physical or emotional, but how much of each." That is a powerful concept that every physician—and anyone with an illness or ailment—must grasp. Simply stated, if we ignore the emotional side, we're not going to be as successful as we could be in getting people better. In my experience, a significant number of doctors fail to appreciate this. So we see more tests, more surgeries, more utilization of our already-strained health-care system—not always to the advantage of the patient. I believe it is one of the key drivers of our out-of-control health (or should I say illness) spending.

Stress, anxiety, depression, and other emotional issues are often the elephant in

SHOULDER THIS

De-Stress

Use relaxation breathing.
ID your stress buttons.
Open your relief valve.
Talk it off.
Soothe yourself.
Think positive.
Eat right and stay hydrated.
Exercise.
Sleep tight.

the corner of the room. Your doctor might see it but might not be comfortable dealing with it. You need to be honest with yourself and bring it up, even if it is only a potential factor. It may be one of the keys to getting you better and/or avoiding unnecessary treatment.

When it comes to psychological distress, clearly there is a wide range of severity. Anyone who is affected daily (work or relationship slippage) by any mind issue must seek professional help. If there are psychosocial issues in play in your case, talk to your doctor about possible interventions. I've heard, and I believe, that broken bodies are easier to heal than broken minds. Addressing the mind is an important step toward optimal healing and recovery, and it's a big part of the Frame-Work program.

STARVE WHATEVER IT IS THAT'S EATING YOU

Doctors aren't the only ones not doing enough when it comes to mind frame—everyone bears some responsibility for how they feel and how that affects health. You may not be able to do much about the circumstances that weigh upon you, but you sure can acknowledge that they exist (don't bury your head in the sand), and you sure can do a lot to combat them.

Use Relaxation Breathing

Unconsciously, most of us take shallow breaths all day long, and that is the rule when we are in pain or in an excited or agitated state, which actually produces or exacerbates stress.

The following routine to calm you down is so simple that you can do it anywhere, anytime, and it's something you should do a few times every day and whenever you are experiencing discomfort or pain.

1. Find a quiet place and get comfortable. Try to relax and let go of tension in your body.

2. Notice your regular breathing—feel it expanding your lungs, then emptying from your lungs.

3. Take deeper breaths and notice how the infusion of additional oxygen clears your head. Focus exclusively on this, driving everything else from your mind.

4. Take even deeper breaths slowly through your nose. Hold for 1 to 2 seconds. Release the air through your mouth while relaxing your entire body. Repeat three times.

5. Breathe normally through your nose three times, focusing on the oxygen coming into your body and thinking about it expanding your chest, entering your bloodstream, and circulating from your forehead to your toes and out to your fingertips.

6. Continue taking slow, deep breaths through your nose, but now let your belly expand so that you're breathing with your diaphragm. When your lungs are full, hold the breath for 2 seconds. (Until you get this deeper breathing down, place your palms on your abdominal area and actually feel your abdomen expand.)

7. Release the breath slowly through your mouth and exhale until your lungs feel completely empty—contract your belly to force out every last air molecule. (If your palms are still on your abdomen, you will feel it deflate and slightly tighten at the end when all the air is exhaled.) Wait 2 seconds.

8. Repeat the cycle three times starting with step 4 above.

Off the Cuff

Right before every intense surgical session, I set aside a few moments to be alone with my breathing. It's something I learned with exposure over the years to martial arts, yoga, and meditation that helps me "cool" my systems. A little time—less than 3 minutes, actually—focusing solely on the air entering and leaving my body, and I'm ready for anything that lies ahead. I'm relaxed, and my concentration is heightened.

ID Your Stress Buttons

There are certain things—at home, at work, at school, even at play—that set your mind and body racing. You usually know what they are (if not, you need to start figuring it out), and you know when they kick in. What you might not know is that you can train yourself to switch off your brain as soon as one of these things occurs: You can make the conscious decision to distract your mind with a more pleasant or innocuous thought. Practice this—it works.

Open Your Relief Valve

You also know what calms you down, distracts you from whatever worries you, and

gets you into the psychological state called flow. Exercise, tennis, and juggling work for me; whatever works for you—a leisurely stroll, model building, poker playing, listening to your playlist, frolicking with the kids—should be brought to the fore whenever you need to let off steam. And although you can't find it in any anatomy book, your funny bone is an essential part of your frame—find it and laugh your cares away every now and then.

Talk It Off

Keeping things bottled up can and will backfire with physical and emotional consequences. Talk to a friend, a significant other, or your doctor. It really helps to let things out. In *FrameWork for the Lower Back*, I cited a recent study published in the *Archives of Internal Medicine* that showed that participation in an e-mail discussion group was enough to help reduce pain and disability in individuals with chronic lower-back pain. There's no reason to think it wouldn't work for shoulder (or mind) pain as well. Talk or chat or text your way to better health.

Soothe Yourself

There is a host of things that pacify just like Mom used to do (or still does, if you're fortunate to still have her with you). Listening to waves at the seashore or staring into a fire (along with other repetitive nature sounds and images); taking a long, hot bath; having a massage; doing yoga, meditation, tai chi, or progressive muscle relaxation (PMR—see below, and combine it with relaxation breathing); and drinking hot tea or water with lemon all have remarkable salutary effects. Take every opportunity you can to nurture your mind frame.

Think Positive

Optimism might not be in your nature, but its proven benefits are so huge that it pays to learn to suspend your disbelief or cynicism. Pick up one or a couple of the bestsellers on

this topic and adopt the approaches and techniques that are most comfortable for you.

Guided imagery (used for centuries by yogis to control heart rate and body temperature) is a form of positive thinking. Studies have shown that an aquarium in a room can lower blood pressure, and that conjuring a tranquil place or activity in your mind can have the same effect. Stay with the image, make it real, and don't be surprised if your tension eases.

Along with the above approaches, here are a few others to keep stress in check.

- Eat right: Food affects mood, as anyone who has witnessed a child after a sugar binge can tell you.

- Hydrate, hydrate, hydrate. (We've discussed how a lack of water can strain your eyes, neck, and back—is it a surprise that these add to overall tension?).

- Stick to an exercise program and get proper sleep.

There are a lot of proven stress reducers to choose from here, but don't let that increase your anxiety. The only must-learn strategy is relaxation breathing, because its calming effect not only cuts tension but prepares your frame for exercise. As for the rest, again,

---

SHOULDER THIS

PMR

In succession:

- Clench and unclench your jaw.
- Shrug your shoulders.
- Make a tight fist and release it.
- Tense and untense your arms, torso, pelvic area, and legs.
- Feel the tension leave your muscles and body.

choose wisely and incorporate everything that's appropriate to your circumstances and preference.

LAST, BUT FIRST

In the previous step you checked your posture. Good form is not just something they used to teach at finishing schools. It's the only way to make sure each of your body parts can do its job properly.

Holding on to the proper alignment is a struggle, I admit, because, in almost all of life, the action is in front of us: We lean forward to see, hear, touch, and connect. And sitting at a desk or behind the wheel of a car (or on a couch watching TV) only makes it

SHOULDER THIS

Posture Tips

SIT UP STRAIGHT! Flatten your lower back into the chair to ensure that you're neither overarching nor rounding at your waist. Pull your shoulders back (imagine your shoulder blades moving toward each other in the midline of your back). Position your seat so that whatever it is you need to see is directly in front of your eyes. The idea is not to have to tilt your head up or down for an extended period of time. Be especially careful at the computer or when relaxing on a couch or armchair.

STAND UP STRAIGHT! But don't lock your knees when you stand. Bend your knees very slightly to prevent your hips from rolling forward. This takes the pressure off your lower back. Imagine there's a string attached to your head that's pulling you upward, as if you were a puppet. Pull your shoulder blades back to square them off so that you could run a straightedge from the back of one shoulder to the other.

MOVE SMARTLY! When walking or running, hold your head high and look toward the horizon, not down. Don't cross your arms in front of you, as that makes your muscles work harder to recenter your torso with every stride.

RELAX RIGHT! When resting, lying in the fetal position on a firm but accommodating mattress is best for your back. Don't tuck a pillow behind your neck, because that can put a crimp in it. Be careful reading or watching TV in bed, as both tend to put the neck in an awkward position (especially with pillows propped behind the head) for extended periods of time.

worse. After a while, your shoulders round, your chin sags, your lower back collapses, and your belly bulges.

Rather than allowing the spine to do its work, poor posture forces your muscles, tendons, and ligaments to support your body. Over time, these soft tissues begin to conform to this out-of-shape shape. Worse, they accept it as the norm and adjust to accommodate. This makes proper form in sports, in dance, and even in walking or running next to impossible.

A slumping spinal column can't do its job as a shock absorber. The disks between vertebrae are meant to absorb the impact of running or jumping by displacing it throughout the spinal column. When you slump, you can't breathe properly, and shabby posture restricts the flow of blood through the muscles, which means there's less of a "flush" to remove metabolic waste, including lactic acid. So it just pools up in your muscles, leading to chronic strain of the neck and the upper and lower back.

As a final check before embarking on the FrameWork shoulder program that follows, look again at the side-view photo you took in Step 3. Most of what it takes to fix any of your imbalances is using the posture tips in the

SHOULDER THIS

Tightness in the front of the shoulder is often a main contributor to poor posture. It not only strains the spinal area and upper back, but is also a setup for a variety of shoulder problems. Tightness can be hard to address, but I have found a simple technique to help:

Stand tall with your shoulders pulled back and your upper back exposed, shirtless if you wish. Have someone place 2-inch surgical-type tape across your upper back and shoulder blade area (where a name would be written on the back of a football jersey). Put your shirt on and try to spend a few hours (or longer) with the tape in place. Whenever you forget and try to slouch forward, the tape will give you a gentle tactile reminder to stand upright. Try this on a regular basis, and it won't take long to break a bad posture habit.

box on page 89 during the day, every day. If you take another photo after just a couple of weeks, you'll be amazed how much better "framed" you are for working out.

ACTIVE SHOULDERS, STEP BY STEP

If you are to extend the warranty on your frame to the fullest, you have to have a healthy lifestyle, balanced fitness, and a mind that's in good shape. In other words: overall health. Paying attention to the approaches above will get you there. If you want to delve into these topics in greater detail, I refer you to my original FrameWork book, *FrameWork—Your 7-Step Program for Healthy Muscles, Bones, and Joints*.

When you have overall health, you minimize the chances of shoulder problems and maximize the benefits of taking the next step that strengthens your entire upper body with targeted exercise. If you don't follow the approaches above, and do them right, you're setting yourself up for "downtime" down the road. I have seen far too many weak, damaged, or injured shoulders exert a domino effect and have a negative impact on individuals' entire lives. This doesn't have to be the case for anyone, regardless of circumstance, who takes the next step.

If your shoulders are tight and creaky now, they'll loosen up and quiet down; if you're a recreational sport enthusiast, you'll play better; if you just want to get out of your car without contorting your upper body, it can be so. Just turn the page to start a whole new chapter in an active life.

SHAPELY SHOULDERS

As we discussed in the previous step, some healthy recommendations never go out of style. The ones I included in other FrameWork books about proper preparation for working out still hold true, and that's how this exercise step starts.

Unfortunately, some of the things they are intended to correct have a habit of hanging around, too, and what I've preached about training throughout the FrameWork book series and in the PBS television special (*Your Body's FrameWork*) bears repeating: Most of my patients are committed to regular exercise, but approximately 80 percent need a modification to their program because it overworks or underworks one or more vulnerable or potentially vulnerable frame parts.

From the most tentative participant to the most seasoned workout fanatic, I often discover that something just isn't right. If people stick to the "generic" program, not the one customized for *their* frame, they will certainly get into trouble if they haven't already. The

satisfaction I get from their efforts is tempered by the worry that they'll injure themselves and discontinue one of the very best things they can do for their health—being active for life.

A major scientific study has shown that one-third of exercisers had to drop out of a very conservative, medically supervised fitness program because a musculoskeletal ailment—a frame injury—cropped up. The researchers were surprised, but I wasn't. So if problems can result under tight supervision, imagine what could happen if you don't go about things the right way. Your regimen might be great on the merits, but it might not be great for *your* frame.

Does it make much sense to sign up for a

marathon if you can't walk to the corner store without difficulty? Of course not. Likewise, it isn't prudent to train your shoulders vigorously if your body and mind aren't in tune for that exercise, if you aren't fit in general. If you have an issue specifically with your shoulders, it is especially important to have your program appropriately customized to keep you on the field or at the gym—and out of my office. (And there is no getting around the previous step—a healthy lifestyle and general fitness—that must be a prelude to the programs designed for your shoulders.)

Before we get to specific exercises, a couple of reminders are critical.

■ Never embark upon a new exercise routine without disclosing your intent to your primary physician and any other appropriate health-care provider, especially someone who is involved in the care of the body part that the routine targets. This is especially true if you have had significant ongoing or recurrent shoulder problems or shoulder surgery. Temper your enthusiasm for getting started with this prudent check beforehand, and if you answer yes to any of the questions in the Physical Activity Readiness Questionnaire, or PARQ (above right)—which was developed in Canada to help individuals

SHOULDER THIS

Physical Activity Readiness Questionnaire (PARQ)

1. Has your doctor ever said that you have a heart condition and that you should engage in physical activity only as recommended by a doctor?

2. Do you feel pain in your chest when you engage in physical activity?

3. In the past month, have you had chest pain when you were not engaging in physical activity?

4. Do you lose your balance because of dizziness, or do you ever lose consciousness?

5. Do you have a bone or joint problem (for example, back, hip, or shoulder) that could be made worse by a change in your physical activity?

6. Is your doctor currently prescribing drugs (for example, water pills) for your blood pressure or heart condition?

7. Do you know of any other reason why you should not engage in physical activity?

determine if they need to see a doctor before starting an exercise program—your phone call will likely result in an appointment for a thorough examination. If you honestly answered no to all the PARQ questions, you can be reasonably sure that you can start becoming much more physically active. (The American College of Sports Medicine [ACSM] offers a more comprehensive pre-exercise screening based on your age, health status, current or past symptoms, and medical risk factors. If you have a sedentary life-style and/or are older than 50, I strongly recommend an ACSM-type assessment, especially if you have medical issues.) Also, if there are a lot of red flags in your Frame-Work shoulder self-test, notably if you have had difficulty or pain with some of the physical tests, check with your orthopaedic surgeon or sports-medicine specialist before jumping into the program.

- Slow, controlled movement, not bouncing to and fro, is the cornerstone of safe and effective exercise routines. And keep in mind there is significant benefit from both concentric (up) and eccentric (down) motion. Optimal, balanced muscle growth and development require attention to both phases of the lift—up and down—whether it is a biceps curl or a shoulder press, because each builds the muscle differently. Both will increase endurance and build strong body parts, so don't cut yourself short when doing your shoulder routines. Also, the exercises to come will be more effective if you use a mindfulness technique that helps you stay focused and concentrate on the muscles that the movements call upon.

Remember: Just because the focus of this book is the shoulder, you cannot neglect the remainder of your body. In fact, for optimal shoulder health and function, the rest of your body needs to be in top shape and running smoothly. Problems in the neck, lower back,

JOINT DISCUSSION

If the shoulder girdle were to be considered an orchestra, then the scapula has been rightfully named the conductor of the shoulder. Proper scapula movement, strength, and function are essential for a happy, pain-free shoulder. When the scapula is not functioning properly, shoulder problems are sure to follow. In addition, every proper shoulder evaluation starts with an assessment of the shoulder blade.

and core, or any weakness in your legs, can manifest itself in shoulder dysfunction. The body compensates, and while that sometimes helps, often it does not and other problems arise. That is the nature of the kinetic chain and biomechanical principles that govern your frame. Terrific total-body programs can be found in my other FrameWork books and many fitness publications, or, better yet, schedule a few sessions with a certified fitness professional at your local gym.

IN THE STARTING BLOCKS

Have you ever noticed how competitive runners do some last-minute stretches and take a few deep breaths right before they get into position for a race? I have. As a physician for professional athletes for many years, I have had the opportunity to arrive at the stadium hours before a sporting match begins, and I can tell you that athletes devote an extensive amount of time to preparing their bodies for what's to come, executing all the movements required for their sport at reduced speed.

Regardless of the sport or recreational exercise, your frame has to be properly prepared if you want to perform better—and avoid injury. Before you dash out the door in running attire, pick up a racket or golf club, hit the gym, or

engage in the targeted exercise that follows, devote a couple of minutes to the relaxation breathing routine outlined in the previous step and to these other two activities that ensure a healthy workout.

CARDIO WARMUP

Again, you have to get your blood moving before you exercise—throughout the body and deep into your shoulder. And the more in shape you get, the more important warming up is: Your body is capable of doing more, and it will tax its frame members more. (Remember, warming up is different from stretching. Warming up brings blood to your muscles, lubricates your joints, and allows your musculoskeletal tissues to behave elastically and thus be less vulnerable.)

Three to 5 minutes of jumping jacks, cycling, power walking, jogging, or marching in place is all it takes. Blood will flow to the nooks and crannies of the shoulder area (and throughout your body), allowing the working tissues to behave more elastically, thus preventing injury. The key is to break a light sweat; do it every time to avoid injury and get the most out of your shoulder exercises.

Next, do some shoulder rolls (lift shoulders upward and slowly roll backward), followed by arm circles, in which you place your arms straight outward and make the letter T with your body as you rotate your arms. (Palms should be facing forward, with hands and elbows at shoulder height.) These are best starting with small circles and going larger and larger. Do 20 with a backward rotation, followed by 20 going forward. If your shoulder is stiff or painful, you may need to stick with smaller circles and/or keep your arms in a more downward position, or even start with pendulum exercises (see page 144).

JOINT DISCUSSION
Watch Out for Overtraining!

Some level of burnout is natural after a steady slog of hard work. Even 8 weeks after a marathon, a runner's muscles are still regenerating, trying to recover, and his immune system is depleted, which makes him more prone to colds and the flu. Exercise is medicine with a dose-response curve: Exercise a little and you boost your immunity; overdose, and it's depleted.

Simple overreaching leads to muscle soreness, decreased coordination, dampened libido, and, often, more frequent sniffles and coughs. What we call tapering, a period of lighter training, will usually cure this. Persistent underperforming—with or without the depression or anxiety that can accompany overreaching—that does not respond to 2 weeks of tapering or rest may be true overtraining. A combination of psychological stress and inadequate recovery time can cause immune suppression, hormonal imbalances, and chronic inflammation. Other symptoms include lethargy, boredom, nagging muscle soreness, and a marked increase in resting heart rate.

Ten to 20 percent of all athletes and 60 percent of elite distance runners fall into overtraining at least once in their careers. Athletes overtrain most when they adopt the regimen of a famous star, train without a coach or partner, or train with athletes who are at a much higher level. In addition, athletes and active individuals on the low-carb bandwagon are particularly susceptible to overtraining blahs. Inadequate fluid intake will also get you into trouble pretty quickly.

JOINT DISCUSSION

Not everyone is a Gumby, and many individuals are strung pretty tight in terms of their flexibility. Proprioceptive neuromuscular facilitation (PNF) is an aid to stretching that's especially effective for stubborn tight areas, "tight" individuals, or those with recurrent muscle pulls.

While there are several varieties used in the world of rehab, I prefer the contract-relax technique. Normally when you stretch a muscle, it reaches a limit; it just won't go any farther without tearing or straining. But when you contract that same muscle prior to the stretch, then hold for about 20 seconds while continuing to tighten, the contraction acts like a circuit breaker, momentarily overriding your muscle-tightening limits and adjusting your stretch reflex, which is determined by your muscles' stretch receptors. When the muscle is relaxed after that contraction, it momentarily has a new "set point" of limitation and is able to safely elongate or lengthen more.

PNF techniques are especially useful in the shoulder region and can be used with any tight muscle group. Try them with the TriSho stretch (page 107), the doorjamb stretch (page 105), or the sleeper stretch (page 151). For example, before you start the TriSho stretch, hold your right elbow with your left hand with the elbow tip pointing upward. Now try to pull your right elbow back down toward your side but don't let it move, resisting the motion with your left hand. Hold this isometric-type contraction for 10 to 20 seconds, relax, and immediately go into the full TriSho stretch.

Chances are you won't need PNF techniques for every muscle group, but most of us could use them for certain stubborn, tight areas. They work especially well when used as a partner stretch, that is, a stretch with someone else's assistance. Before many pro games begin, you will often see athletes lying on the field or court going through some of these maneuvers with their trainers. Your partner, however, needs to be careful not to force any movement.

SHOULDER THIS

Tennis is my passion, and if I didn't adhere to the following routine religiously, I'd be on the sidelines a lot more.

- 30 jumping jacks
- Jogging in place or shadowboxing-type movements
- Rotational twists
- Side bends
- Toe touching
- Deep knee bends (I have to hold on to something because of a cranky knee.)
- Shoulder, forearm, and calf stretching
- Holding my racket, I go through tennis-specific movement patterns to awaken muscle memory: windmills, low-intensity service motion, and practice swings (starting in slow motion and gradually increasing the pace, all while using the visualization technique to hone my shots).
- Gentle volleying from midcourt for a couple of minutes

I spend a scant 5 minutes off the court and about the same on it. In less than 10 minutes, I'm good to go.

S-T-R-E-T-C-H

This is a great idea anytime; it's indispensable before a workout. For those of you who are strung particularly tight, try to stretch every day and follow the 3 x 20 stretching routine, holding each stretch below for 20 seconds and repeating three times. The shoulder area is particularly prone to developing tight, contracted areas, often without your even being aware of it. Regular shoulder stretching will prevent this common problem. For athletes or those involved in sports, additional dynamic stretches (such as arm swings and other joint rotations) can also be helpful and should be incorporated. Also, consider taking up yoga and get a copy of *Stretching* by Bob Anderson (Shelter Publications), or my original Frame-Work book.

Remember: Your shoulders are connected to the rest of your frame, and every part must work in concert. You reap maximum reward when stretching routines precede every frame workout (after you've broken a sweat with a cardio warmup, of course).

PROGRAM YOUR SHOULDERS

The FrameWork "Active for Life" shoulder routine falls into three broad areas:

- Basic Shoulder Training (to keep healthy shoulders healthy) (starting on this page)

- Neuromuscular and High Performance Training (for the high-performance shoulder) (see page 131)

- Recovery and Rehabilitation (for the problem shoulder) (see page 142)

First and foremost, if you've had shoulder surgery recently or you have a balky shoulder, the **Recovery and Rehab** programs are where you should begin getting your shoulders back in shape. (But don't skip reading the **Basic Shoulder Training** below, because that's what you'll be doing soon enough—once your shoulders are healthy or asymptomatic and you want to keep them that way. You may even be able to incorporate some of the basic exercises right from the start.)

The Basic Shoulder Training program works all the primary shoulder muscles—deltoid, trapezius, rhomboid, serratus, rotator cuff, and scapular area (see sidebar)—and the core muscles that work in conjunction with them. This comprehensive exercise routine is divided into three sections:

- Flexibility
- Strength
- Core and More

SHOULDER THIS

Shoulder health starts on the floor and goes through the core.

Start with the first exercise in each area and add the next one when you are comfortable enough to do so. For many of the specific body parts, I offer a variety of exercise options, including ones that can be done at home (with minimal if any equipment) or at the gym. Pick one or two that target each muscle group—no need to do them all. Don't worry if you can do only certain ones at the start, or if one area is problematic for you. Each person has a unique set of circumstances related to body weight, overall fitness, and health issues, and your frame will be introduced to exercises it hasn't experienced yet. There is no timetable for getting to all of them; just work steadily at your own pace while keeping the goal of being able to do all of them (someday) in mind.

BASIC SHOULDER TRAINING PROGRAM

The comprehensive routine that follows contains quite a number of individual exercises, but if you're a FrameWork veteran, you are already doing many of them. If you aren't, you'll find that once you get the hang of a shoulder workout, it will be easy to incorporate into your regular nonaerobic workouts.

Don't fret if a piece of equipment isn't available or if you can't do every exercise at the start. If you go to a gym, you can find machines that will accomplish much of what we are recommending. If you work out at home and want to use strength equipment, a single multitrainer like that pictured in this book is perfect and takes up little room. All the strength exercises can also be performed with some simple, inexpensive portable items, such as elastic bands or tubing and exercise balls that you can get from spri.com. (See the Additional Resources section at the end of the book.)

If your shoulders are healthy and you can work hard, to fatigue, you shouldn't need more than one or two sets two or three times a week—usually not on consecutive days, so that your muscles have time to recover from

JOINT DISCUSSION

Home gyms and workout aids have exploded onto the scene in recent years. If cost and/ or space limitations are a factor, you still have plenty of good options available. The Total Gym is compact and ideally suited to the shoulders and upper body. There are some great multigyms like the Nautilus Freedom Trainer and other "functional trainers" with high/low adjustable cable systems and weight stacks that can target your shoulders (and other joints) from multiple angles.

Regardless of where you go, do your homework first. Get advice from those in the know and *always* try a piece of equipment before you buy. In fact, try it a few times on different days; sometimes it takes your body a day or two to decide if it likes something or not. Even worse, you may have found a weak link and irritated things.

Your height, weight, fitness, and training goal are all unique to you and critical in making a decision. Be sure to discuss this topic with your doctor or a qualified therapist or trainer before making a purchase, and make sure you buy from someone who knows how important individual circumstances are.

the hard workout. To challenge yourself more, perform many of the exercises while seated on a stability ball. This forces you to recruit additional muscles and enhance control of your upper body and torso. In terms of rehabilitation, because you are usually working with lighter loads initially, you will need to perform more sets of exercises, and you will probably be doing them every day and even several times per day. Doing rehab exercises while seated on the stability ball also provides tremendous benefits.

Keep in mind that if you don't work your

shoulders on a regular basis, you won't be getting the most out of your frame—and you'll be setting yourself up for problems down the road. This is true for everyone, from couch potatoes to high-level athletes, and especially true for those whose work or sport places high demands on the shoulder and arm.

JOINT DISCUSSION

There's both good and bad pain during exercise. When you feel "the burn" build gradually during a workout, you're experiencing what has been termed immediate muscle soreness (IMS), which is caused by the buildup of lactic acid and other metabolic wastes in the muscles. There's no harm in this—it's one of the side effects of a really productive workout, and this "good pain" will go away shortly after exercise. Delayed-onset muscle soreness (DOMS) is another type of muscle ache that typically occurs 1 to 2 days after a hard workout, especially a "negative" or eccentric muscle workout, or if you are unaccustomed to weight lifting or are just getting back to it after a layoff.

The time to worry is when you feel sensations such as stinging, stabbing, sharp pain, or tingling numbness instead of a healthy burn. *Stop* what you're doing. You should never have sudden or deep, lasting pain that interferes with sleep, nor should you ever note bruising, swelling, or loss of mobility. All of these sensations could be signs of deeper problems in the shoulder socket or surrounding areas and should be evaluated by a physician.

Neck Roll

To improve neck range of motion

This routine is a variation on the original neck roll that was thought to place undue strain on the neck. It includes gaining neck mobility in three planes: flexion/extension, rotation, and lateral bending. Standing with your arms at your sides, look up, then down; then look to your right, and finally look forward and tilt your head to your right. Now look to your left, and then look forward and tilt your head to your left. Hold each extended position for 5 seconds.

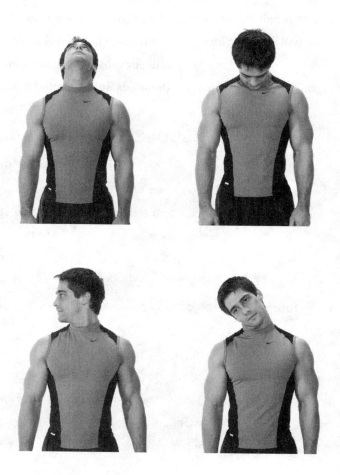

Pillar Stretch

To improve shoulder mobility and rotator cuff function

Interlace your fingers in front of you, then turn your palms outward and reach straight for the ceiling, palms up, until your hands are directly over your head with your elbows straight. Hold for 5 seconds.

Advanced modification:
Alternate leaning gently to your left and right during the hold.

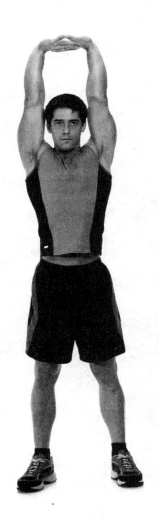
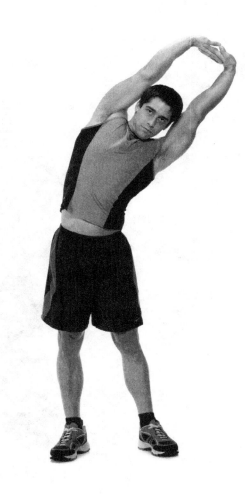

Arm Cross

Improves rear shoulder and rotator cuff flexibility

Fully straighten your left arm in front of you and place your right hand above your left elbow. Using your right arm, pull your left arm across your chest so your forearm is hitting toward your right shoulder. Go until you can't go any farther (you should feel a stretch behind your left shoulder) and hold for 10 seconds. Don't let your elbow drop down; stay high, just below your chin. Then, keeping your arm in this stretched position, let your left elbow flex so you give yourself a hug or a pat on the back. As you improve, you should be able to reach farther across your back. Alternate sides.

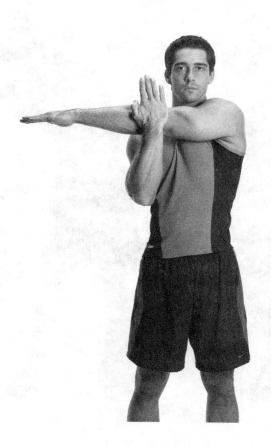

Doorjamb Stretch

Reduces tightness in the front part of the shoulder and pectoral area

This fast and easy routine should be done regularly, even on days when you are not in the gym. The key is to keep your elbow at the same height as your shoulder, and when you lean inward into the open doorway, picture yourself leading with the front of the shoulder arching inward. Keep your palm open and holding the doorjamb (you should feel a stretch in the front of the shoulder). Hold the position for 10 seconds. Switch to the other arm and repeat.

Modification: If you have tight shoulders, motion loss in your shoulders, or rotator cuff issues, consider the towel-stretch alternative: Hold a small towel behind you. Use the towel to first pull your raised arm downward (improves external rotation) and then use the raised arm to pull the lowered one upward (improves internal rotation). Alternate arms.

Alternate: Sit or stand tall and gently clasp your fingers behind your neck, elbows pointing upward. Slowly pull your elbows back while tightening your shoulder blades toward each other. (You should feel a stretch in the front of your shoulders.) Hold for 5 to 7 seconds and relax. Repeat several times.

Note: If you have a shoulder that "pops out" (i.e., dislocates or subluxes anteriorly), **do not** perform these front shoulder stretches.

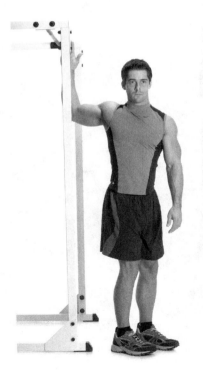
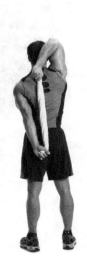
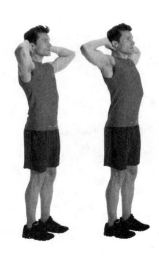

Climb the Rope

For shoulder, latissimus, and spinal mobility

While looking up slightly, tighten your abdominal area (suck it in). Reach way up with your left hand, then reach even higher; cross your right hand over your left as if you were climbing a rope (really reaching is important). You should feel it in your shoulders and upper back. Done correctly, this is excellent for posture and works the entire spinal area and abdominal obliques for both strength and flexibility. Do 5 repetitions on each side.

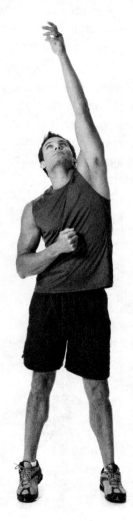

TriSho Stretch

To stretch the triceps and shoulder area as well as the upper lats, reach your right arm up and behind you, patting yourself on the upper back. Now use your left hand to grab your right elbow and gently pull your elbow in toward your head, allowing your right hand to reach farther down your back over your left shoulder blade. Hold for 10 seconds and switch sides.

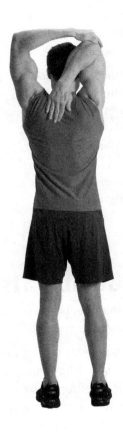

Forearm Stretch

For wrist, forearm, and elbow flexibility, especially for golfers and tennis players or anyone with elbow and/or wrist issues.

Extend your right arm straight in front of you. Let your wrist drop downward. Keeping your fingers straight, use your left hand to push downward on the top of your right hand until your wrist is flexed downward at a 90-degree angle. Hold for 10 seconds. Switch hands and repeat.

Next, keeping your right arm straight, extend your right wrist upward (policeman's stop). Use your left hand to pull back your fingers, thumb, and right palm simultaneously so that your wrist is extended upward 90 degrees and your fingers are fully straight or even bent backward a little if possible. Switch arms, and then repeat on each side again. Shake out both hands for a few seconds.

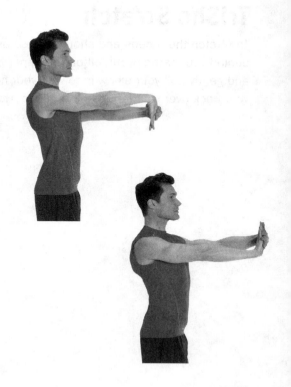

Forearm/Pillar Combo Stretch

A fast, simple dynamic stretch that can be done anytime—great if you've been sitting at your desk or computer for extended periods.

Start with your hands clasped, arms straight outward in front of you, palms facing inward and wrists flexed so that you're making a 90-degree angle at the wrists. Push outward as far as you can, feeling a stretch in your outer forearms and rear shoulders. Hold for 5 to 7 seconds. Next, flip your hands so your palms are facing outward, hands still clasped, and again push outward, fully straightening your elbows. Hold for 5 to 7 seconds.

Holding your elbows straight, slowly raise your arms upward into the pillar stretch position (page 103), palms facing upward, directly over your head. Hold for 5 to 7 seconds, pushing your palms upward as high as you can. Repeat the entire sequence three times. (A quicker version of this stretch, which I call 3-2-1, Touch the Sun, involves the same sequence, but you hold each position only momentarily.)

Child's Pose

For spine and shoulder mobility

Start in a kneeling position. Gently rock back onto your heels (or as far as you can comfortably go). Lower your forehead and chest area toward the floor as your arms (palms down) reach forward. Slide your palms forward as far as they will go, feeling both a relaxation and a stretch in the spine, latissimus, and shoulder area. Breathe slowly and deeply while relaxing your arms, shoulders, and upper back. Hold for 5 seconds.

Standing modification (if you have back, hip, or knee problems): Lean forward along a Smith machine or countertop with your arms straight out while bending at the waist and looking downward. Gently rock your hips and pelvis backward so that you feel a stretch in the upper-back, lat, and shoulder area.

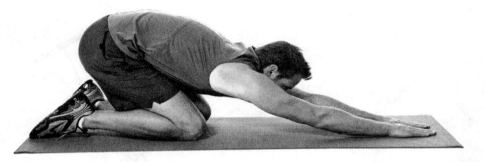

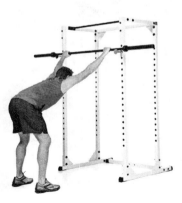

Lat Pulldown

Builds a strong upper back and V shape; also helps prevent shoulder problems

This can be done with a wide grip, palms out; or a more narrow grip, palms in (my preference); or one arm at a time (with tubing or pulley). As you pull down, there is a tendency to lean back; slight leaning is okay, but don't use the momentum of leaning back to assist the movement, because that cheats the lats. Slowly bring the bar to your breastbone area and concentrate on using your lats to do the work. (As a side note, I don't like the behind-the-neck lat pulldown, which all too often irritates the neck and shoulder areas.)

Alternates: The free-weight version is the single-arm dumbbell row, and the tubing version is a tubing lat pulldown. Also, chinups are a great alternative and can be done as "negative" chinups—starting in the up position with some assistance, then lowering yourself slowly on your own.

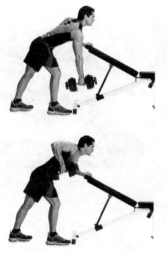

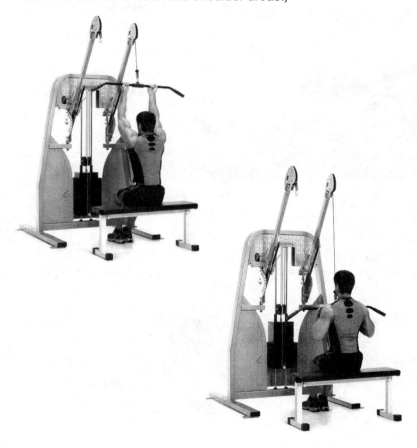

Machine Row

Improves posture and is important for rotator cuff health and function

If you are doing this properly, you don't need much weight. The body cheats by bringing in momentum (by moving too fast) and also by having your elbows drop slightly down, which brings in your lats rather than working the rear shoulder, rear cuff, and scapular (shoulder blade) stabilizer.

Keep your elbows high (at shoulder level throughout the entire movement) and lean backward with your elbow tips, imagining strings attached to your elbows, pulling them backward. You should feel the muscles working behind your shoulders and around your shoulder blades. (Another version of this exercise can be done with elastic tubing and a tubing door attachment.)

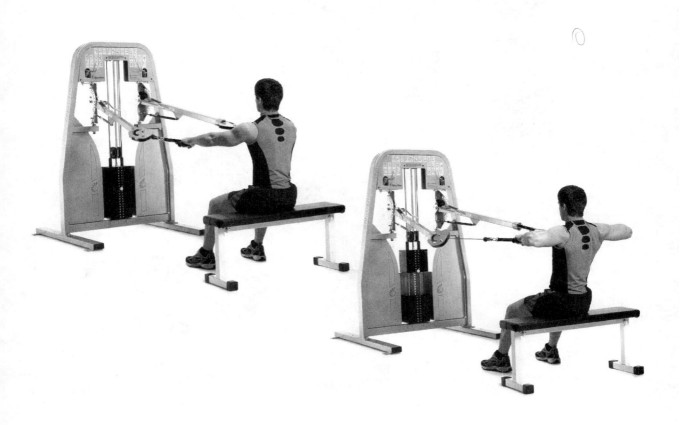

Single-Arm Dumbbell Rear Cuff Row

This exercise really targets the rear deltoid and the rear shoulder area, which is often neglected. Lean on a bench with your left hand, keeping your back flat. Don't bob up and down. Your right elbow and arm should be the only things moving. Keeping the elbow at the same level as the shoulder (not dropping downward), lead with your elbow upward. Imagine a string pulling the elbow toward the ceiling.

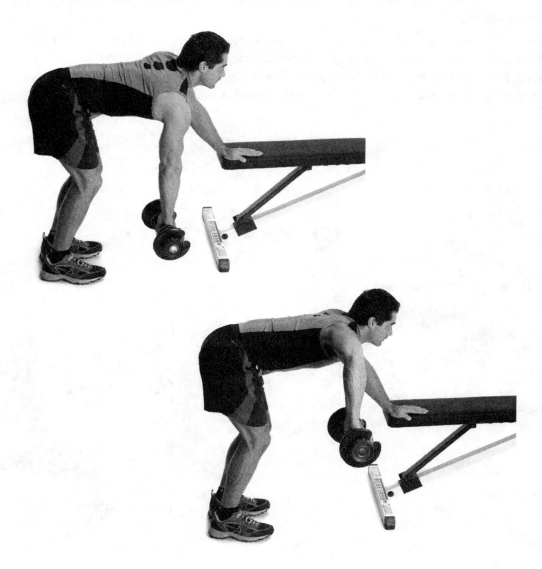

Bow and Arrow

Hold elastic tubing tightly with your left arm extended and your right hand in front of your chest. Keeping your right elbow higher than your right shoulder, pull back on the tubing with your right hand but actually feel the motion lead from your right elbow heading backward. Pull until you are in the fully extended position as if you were squeezing your shoulder blades together, also pulling both shoulders backward. Your left hand and right elbow should be slightly behind the plane of your shoulders, and you should feel a slight stretch in the chest area. (Use extremely light tubing if you have any shoulder problems.) Switch sides and repeat.

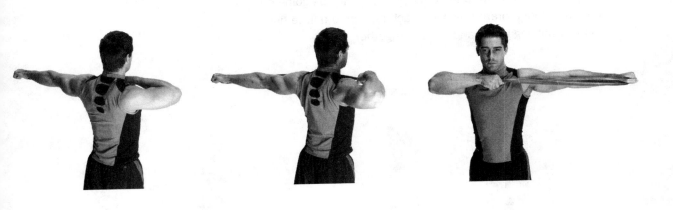

JOINT DISCUSSION
Rotator Cuff Strengthening

The basic shoulder program outlined here will go a long way toward strengthening your shoulder, including your rotator cuff muscles. However, as I have mentioned earlier in the book, the rotator cuff group of muscles is small and relatively difficult to isolate and optimally strengthen. If you have had shoulder difficulties or if your sport or work demands much more of your shoulders, then you should add the specific rotator cuff strengthening exercises (pages 153 and 154) to this standard shoulder routine, and don't forget to try them while seated on a stability ball for added benefits. (Ditto for the "high-performance" shoulder.)

Upright Row

Stand facing a machine, holding onto the handle, arms straight down with palms facing inward. Using your shoulders, slowly lift upward until your hands are just below your chin. Pause for a moment and slowly lower the weight to the starting position. Keep your neck relaxed, avoiding the tendency to tighten it backward, especially if you have neck problems. There is a tendency, especially if you're lifting too much weight, to tighten and compress the neck area. If you have shoulder problems, keep the weight lower and do the first 3 or 4 reps going only to the breastbone area; then with each rep come a little higher. Also try moving your hands closer together.

Alternates: The free-weight version can be with a barbell or tow dumbbells. The tubing version can be done while standing on the elastic tubing.

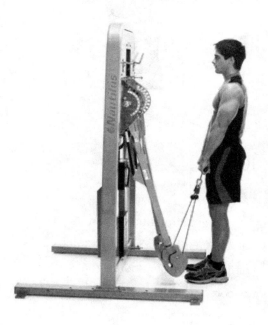
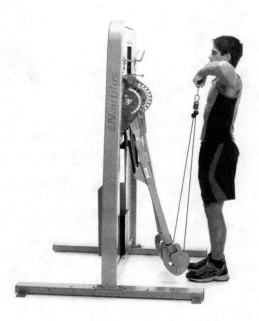

Lateral Raise

Hold dumbells in both hands. Keeping your elbows slightly bent, slowly raise your arms outward until they're parallel to the floor or slightly higher (don't force them too high). As you lift, slightly tilt the thumb sides of your hands downward (as if you're pouring out a little water from a bottle). This better isolates the mid- and rear deltoids and rotator cuffs (the front deltoids get plenty of work with other upper-body exercises; in fact, they're often overworked). Pause, then slowly lower the weights to the starting point. Don't tighten your neck, pulling it back during the lift, which causes neck strain.

Modification: If you have shoulder or neck problems, do this exercise on a machine or with tubing or free weights one arm at a time while supporting yourself. Do not lift as high, and stay just below 90 degrees, keeping your hand below the level of your shoulder until this gets more comfortable. Go higher gradually as tolerated. (If your upper-body problems make this modified version impossible to do, focus more time and effort on the rotator cuff rotation exercises and plan in the Rehab section on pages 153 and 154.)

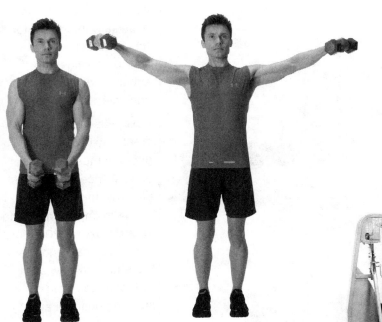

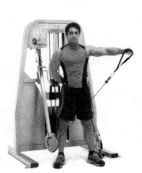

Pec Machine or Barbell Press

Don't arch your back or lift your buttocks off the bench. Don't bounce the weights off your chest. It may feel good and allow you to use more weight, but it can be dangerous to your shoulders, resulting in either a sudden injury or, more common, low-grade cumulative damage over time. Don't lock out your elbows (especially suddenly). Be sure to tighten your abdominal area during the lift, and don't hold your breath. (If you have lower-back problems, it helps to rest your feet on the bench with your knees flexed.)

Modification: If you have shoulder problems, try different angles (i.e., incline or decline) or vary the grip on the barbell. A wider grip works more of the chest area, and a narrower grip works more of the triceps. Vary to find what's comfortable for you. Also, use a pec machine if available and "pin the stack" so your arm doesn't go back as far. This is especially important for those with shoulder instability who either sublux or dislocate their shoulders.

Note: Pushups are another great way to build your pectoral muscles as well as your triceps. Done properly, they also help build the important scapular area. Try for 20 pushups. If you can't do them the standard way, start with pushups from a kneeling position and gradually build up as you can. If they get too easy, challenge yourself with versions shown in the Neuromuscular Training section (page 132).

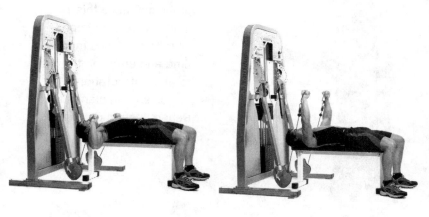

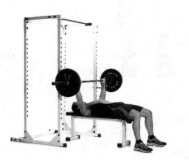

Biceps Curl

Whether you use dumbbells or a barbell, raise the weight slowly, pausing at the top and letting the weight down slowly in a controlled motion. Don't arch your back to help (cheat) with the lift. With dumbbells, start with the weights at your sides, palms inward; alternate arms, and as you get halfway up the lift, supinate slowly so your palm is facing upward at the end of the lift to better contract your biceps. Do 3 sets of 10 repetitions. (If you have lower-back problems, try seated biceps curls with dumbbells.)

Alternates: A standing biceps curl using the upper cable of a machine isolates your biceps nicely and helps develop your biceps "peak." Curls can also be done while standing on tubing, or try them while seated on a stability ball.

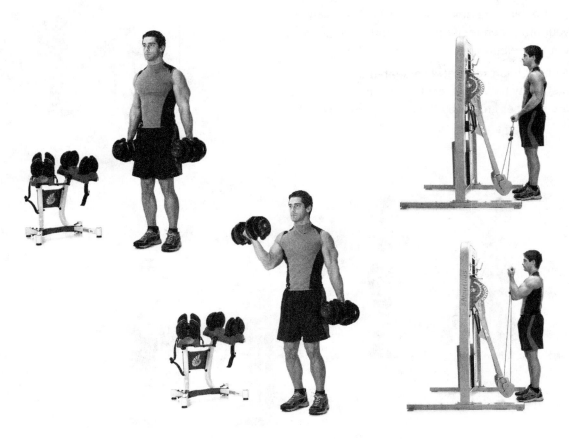

Triceps Extension

As circumstances or preferences dictate, triceps extensions can be done using a single-arm kickback supported on a bench (at right), a rope-pulley-cable triceps extension (below), or an elastic-tubing pulldown or kickback.

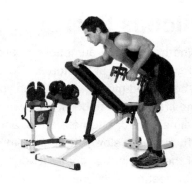

Move the weights slowly into full extension so you can squeeze and fully contract the triceps. Do not suddenly "lock out" your elbow; rather, slowly squeeze the motion until your elbow is straight. (If you have elbow problems, especially pain behind the elbow when you fully straighten your arm, then resist the temptation to fully lock out your elbows.)

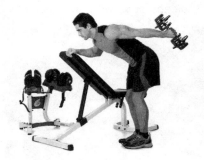

Also try this exercise while seated on a stability ball. Slow, controlled dips are another great way to build your triceps.

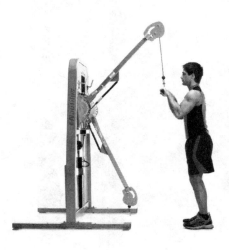

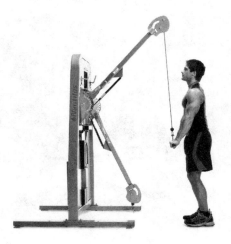

Forearm Curls

Forearm strengthening starts with a light dumbbell, elastic tubing, or weighted pulley (see photo). Do 10 wrist curls (palm up) with each hand, followed by reverse wrist curls (palm down) with each hand. There are also many hand-grip strengtheners that are helpful for strong grip and forearm strength as well as injury prevention. Keep one at your desk at work or in your nightstand for daily use.

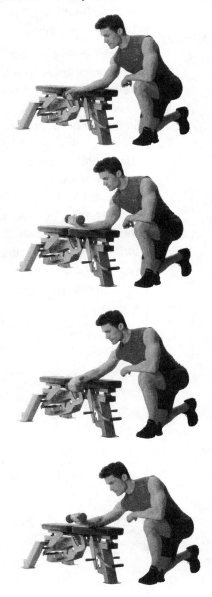

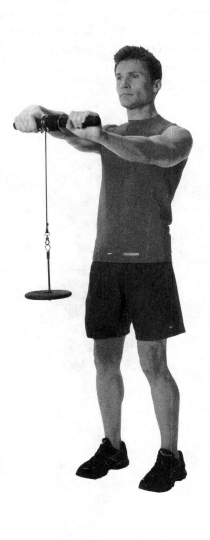

Stork

To improve balance

Stand up straight, extend your arms out wide to your sides, and raise your left foot off the floor to the level of your right knee. Rest the arch of your left foot on the inner side of your right knee, forming the letter P. Try not to sway or rock to maintain balance. Hold for 10 seconds on each foot; try to build up to 20 seconds. (This is a good time to practice your relaxation breathing as you exercise.)

Advanced version: As this gets easier, try to perform it with your eyes closed, on the ball of your foot, or on a small, firm pillow (or wobble board or BOSU trainer, if available).

Note: This is a simple way to improve balance and will help with injury and fall prevention as well as improve sports performance. If you have had an injury (especially to a knee, foot, or ankle) this may be difficult, but it is an important part of your total recovery. If you have difficulty with this exercise, you should perform it several times a day, every day.

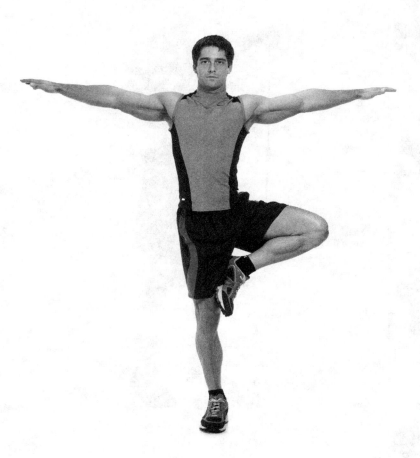

Crunch

Lie on the floor, knees bent and feet flat. Start with a pelvic tilt maneuver, tightening your abs. Do not throw yourself forward. Do not clasp your hands behind your head, but keep them near your ears or across your chest. Do not anchor your feet under anything or have someone hold your feet, as this allows you to use your hip flexor muscles rather than your abs.

Tighten your abdominal muscles and slowly curl your head and shoulders off the floor; feel your breastbone accordion in toward your upper pubic bone. Don't come up past 30 degrees, as you would in an old-fashioned situp. Keep your lower back on the floor and don't use your hands to pull your neck or head forward. Pause momentarily; then, very slowly, in a controlled manner, come back down. Slowly exhale during the lifting phase and inhale during the lowering phase. You should feel the movement, the "burn," in your abs. Concentrate on the feeling in your abs and not on how high you can rise. Do 20 reps. (Add more each day as you get better.)

Note: In most gyms, there are great machine options for total abdominal work, and they include the ab machines or machine crunch as well as the rotary torso for obliques. There are also numerous alternatives that are worth incorporating into your workouts at various times. The basic crunch tends to work the upper abdominal area. To target your lower abdominal area, do a hanging shoulder raise from a chinup bar or do a reverse crunch, in which you keep your head and shoulders on the floor and slowly bring your hips upward, then downward.

Advanced version—crunch with a twist: Lie on your back with your ankles crossed and your hips and knees flexed at 90-degree angles. Slowly perform a crunch, bringing your right elbow to your left knee. Hold for 3 seconds. Do 10 repetitions and repeat on the opposite side. (For a slightly easier version, lie on your back with your right knee bent and foot resting on the floor. Cross your left leg over your right knee, keeping your left arm out on the floor. Place your right hand near your right ear and slowly twist up, bringing your right elbow toward your left knee.)

More advanced version: Perform the crunch exercises on a stability ball.

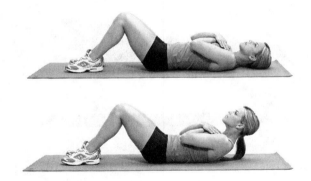

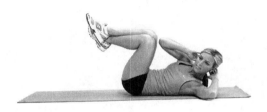

Bird Dog

Start on the floor on all fours. Slowly lift your left arm and right leg simultaneously, holding both straight for 5 to 7 seconds. Do not raise your arm or leg above horizontal; instead, stay parallel to the floor. Then switch sides.

Modified version: If the full bird dog is too difficult, or if you have significant discomfort, try raising only one arm or one leg at a time, and gradually build up to where you can hold both out, even if they are only partially rather than fully raised.

Advanced version: Using ankle weights and a small hand weight, add 3 to 5 pounds per limb.

More advanced version: Start in the "up" position of a pushup. Holding that up position, lift your right arm and left leg simultaneously and hold for 5 to 7 seconds, then switch sides.

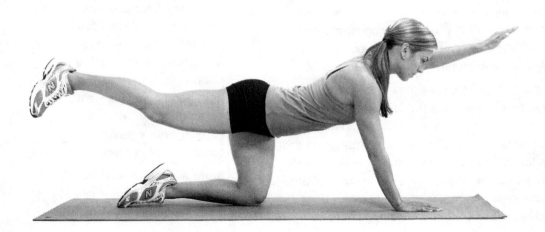

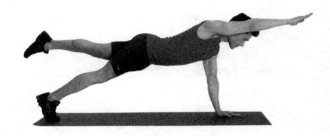

Warrior

Standing and looking straight ahead, balance on your left leg while slowly lifting your right leg backward and extending your arms forward. Bend forward until you feel a stretch in the hamstring of your left leg. Balance on your left leg, forming a T with your body. Keep your back flat and avoid twisting. Hold for 20 to 30 seconds while breathing comfortably. Switch legs and repeat.

Advanced version: As this gets easier, try to perform it with your eyes closed.

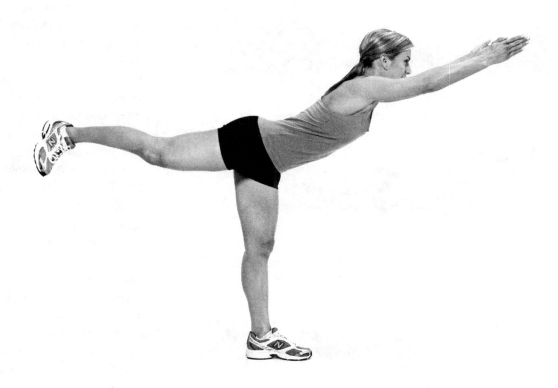

Superman

I first described this exercise almost 30 years ago both to assess spinal strength and to help individuals rebuild their lower backs after injury. It is terrific for spinal extensor muscle strength and maintaining overall spine health.

Lie on the floor facedown with your arms straight out in line with your legs. (Picture Superman flying in the air.) Simultaneously bring both arms and both legs off the floor. Only your abdominal area and pelvis should be touching the floor. Hold for 10 seconds and build up to 20. Do 10 reps.

Advanced version: Simultaneously bring both arms and both legs off the floor. Only your abdominal area and pelvis should be on the floor. Hold for 10 seconds and build up to 20 seconds. Repeat 3 times.

Modified version: If the above is too difficult or causes too much discomfort, raise your left arm and right leg off the floor. Keep your shoulder straight so that your leg is being lifted by your buttocks and lower back. If it doesn't bother your neck, your head should also come off the floor. Hold for 10 seconds and build up to 20. Repeat with your right arm and left leg. Do 3 reps on each side. (If you have neck problems, you can keep your face resting on the floor and not lift your head. If you are unable to do even this version, you can start with lifting only one arm or leg off the floor and build up as tolerated.)

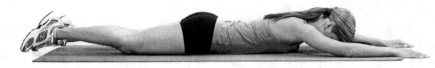

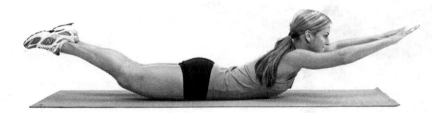

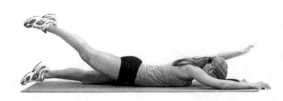

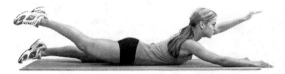

Superman on Ball

This exercise is for spinal extensor and gluteal muscle strength and endurance.

Lie facedown on a stability ball with your toes touching the floor and your arms stretched out in front, reaching forward. Let your spine and entire body relax. Hold for 20 to 30 seconds or as long as you like if you find this comfortable. This is a good lower-back stretch and relaxation exercise and is good to do before starting the actual Superman movement.

Keeping your feet on the floor and your legs straight, slowly extend your lumbar area until your lower back is straight or slightly extended and your arms are fully extended beyond your head, like Superman flying. Hold for 10 seconds and build up to 20 seconds. Do 5 to 10 reps.

To better isolate the rear shoulder area, try the Y version in which you widen your arms outward with your thumbs pointing upward (see photo).

More advanced version: Get into the Superman position and then gently lift one straight leg off the floor, balancing only on the opposite straightened leg. Hold for 5 seconds, then alternate legs.

Most advanced version: Do the full Superman, in which only your abdominal area is on the ball and both feet and arms are outward in the "flying" position. Your feet should be off the floor.

Modified version: If you are unable to perform this move, start by assisting yourself, keeping your hands on the floor and just slightly lifting them off the floor when possible. Gradually build up to where you can straighten your back fully, then start bringing your hands upward to the full Superman.

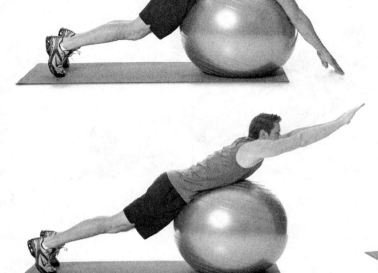

Glute Bridge (with Leg Up)

Lie on the floor with your knees bent at 90 degrees, your feet flat on the floor hip-width apart, and your arms away from your body at 45-degree angles, resting on the floor to support you. Tighten your abs and lift (or bridge) your hips toward the ceiling while tightening your glutes (buttock muscles). Now slowly extend your left leg so that it is straight out, toes pointing toward the ceiling. Hold your left leg out for 5 seconds and then lower it, maintaining the firm bridge position at all times throughout this exercise until all reps are completed. Repeat with your right leg. Complete 10 reps with each leg.

Modified version: If it's too difficult to raise your leg, perform the basic glute bridge with both feet resting on the floor.

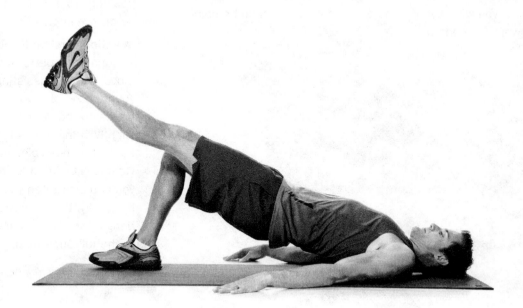

Glute Bridge on Ball

Lie on the floor with your heels on a stability ball and toes pointing upward, arms and palms resting flat on the floor slightly away from your body. Tighten your glutes, lifting your pelvis upward to form a straight line. Only your head, shoulders, and arms will be on the floor. Hold for 3 seconds and slowly drop back down to the floor. Repeat 5 times.

Advanced version: Try crossing your arms in front of your chest, making balance more difficult.

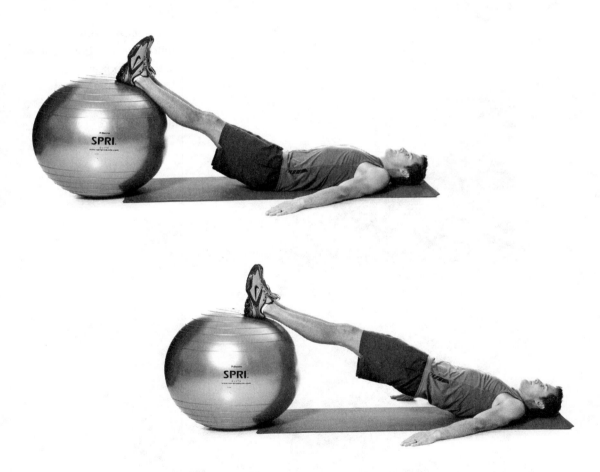

Side Plank on Floor

Lie on your right side with your right forearm and elbow on the floor. Your elbow should be in line with your shoulder, and your torso sagging toward the floor. Lean on your forearm, lifting your hips and shoulders upward into a straight, rigid line while supporting all your weight on your forearm and the side of your right foot. Hold for 20 seconds. Repeat twice and then perform the exercise again, lying on your left side.

Alternate version: Instead of stacking one foot directly on the other, try performing this plank with the foot of the top leg also resting on the floor just in front of your other foot.

Advanced version: Try to increase your hold time to 1 to 2 minutes. If this gets too easy, hold a light weight against the hip that's on top.

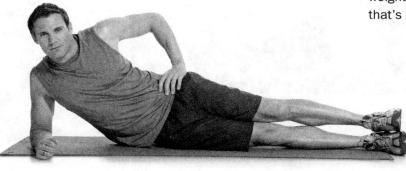

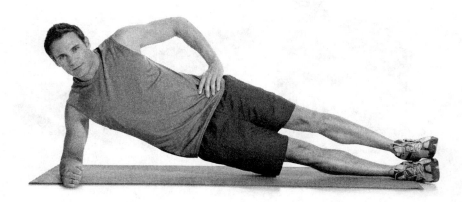

Bridge/Plank on Ball

Rest your elbows and forearms on a stability ball. Tighten your abs and lift upward into the plank position so that your back and legs form a straight line and you are supported only on your elbows and feet. Hold for 20 seconds, keeping your abs and torso area tightened and stabilized. Repeat twice. Try to build up to 1 minute.

Advanced version: Once you are stabilized and secure, slowly lift your left leg in a straight line using your gluteal muscles. Hold for 20 seconds and then change legs. Repeat twice with each leg.

More advanced versions— "body saw" and "stir the pot": In the plank position, gently rock back and forth (just a few inches) on your elbows in a "sawing" motion. Next, try short circular motions, 5 clockwise and 5 counterclockwise, keeping your body straight and not rotating your core area.

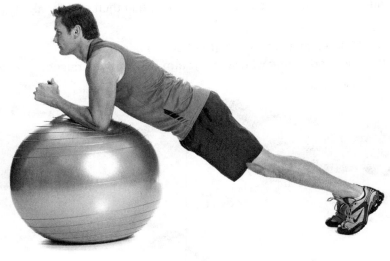

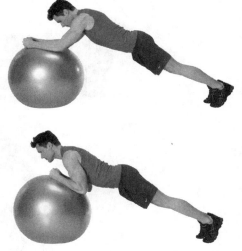

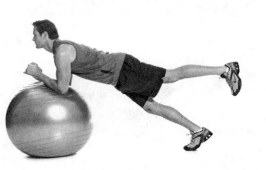

Quadruped

Kneel on the floor and place your forearms flat on the floor as if you were going to do a modified pushup. Now assume the plank position, with your body straight and your full weight supported on both forearms and your toes (first photo). Your body should be straight as a board with your pelvis tucked inward, tightening your abdominal muscles. Try holding this position with your weight on your forearms and toes for 60 seconds.

Now lift your right arm off the floor for 15 seconds, supporting your full weight on your left forearm and both feet (second photo). Switch arms and repeat.

With both forearms on the floor, raise your right leg, hold for 15 seconds, and then repeat, lifting your left leg (not shown).

Next, try to elevate your right arm and left leg simultaneously (third photo) and hold for 15 seconds, then return them to the floor and repeat with your left arm and right leg raised.

Return to the plank position and hold for 30 seconds.

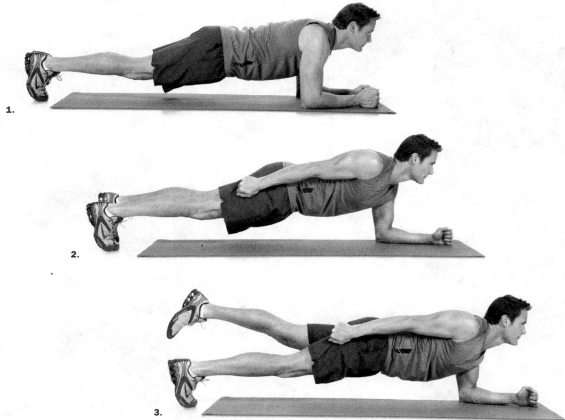

1.

2.

3.

NEUROMUSCULAR AND HIGH-PERFORMANCE TRAINING

The shoulder-specific routines that follow are more advanced than what we have presented so far and are more suitable for individuals whose shoulders and upper bodies demand high performance.

A high-performance shoulder requires much more than just a strong, flexible, balanced shoulder girdle. Remember: The kinetic chain starts at the floor, goes through the legs, hips, and pelvis; passes through the core; and then progresses to the shoulders and arm area. I particularly like the two exercises (single-leg squat and tic-tac-toe bunny hop) on pages 139 and 140, but they are by no means all you need for a strong, durable base. Regularly do the core exercises that start on page 120. Include comprehensive lower-body strengthening and stretching, especially hip abductions and adductions, leg extensions, leg curls, lunges, squats, and calf raises. Also include lower-body agility, proprioception, and plyometrics. Basic and advanced routines can be found in both *FrameWork for the Knee* and *FrameWork for the Lower Back*, and they include modifications for those with knee and lower-back problems. I cannot emphasize enough how important a strong core and strong legs are for healthy, high-performance shoulders. (For more neuromuscular training information, see Additional Resources on page 195.)

JOINT DISCUSSION

Neuromuscular training has taken center stage in the world of sports performance and injury prevention. It started with many creative routines for the core and lower body and now has found its way to the shoulder region. There are numerous techniques, including plyometrics and other agility drills, designed for this purpose, and the programs continue to evolve. I include some sample routines but also urge readers to do more research and talk to their orthopaedic surgeons, therapists, and trainers for more specific, individualized instruction. Every athlete, at all ages, should be involved in these preventive training programs. Parents and coaches must take a more proactive stance in this regard, and I remain baffled by the fact that such programs aren't being offered routinely in schools and on playing fields across the country.

Pushup with Medicine Ball and Stability Ball

Pushups can be performed with one or both hands on a medicine ball. To make things more challenging once you are fully up, bring the opposite hand (the one not on the medicine ball) to your chest for 2 to 3 seconds. Practice this in the modified pushup position on your knees until you're able to do the full pushup. Another alternative is to perform the pushups with both hands on a stability ball. To make this more challenging, cross your ankles or lift a leg up so that you are supported on only one leg. If this is too difficult, practice in the modified pushup position, on your knees instead of your toes.

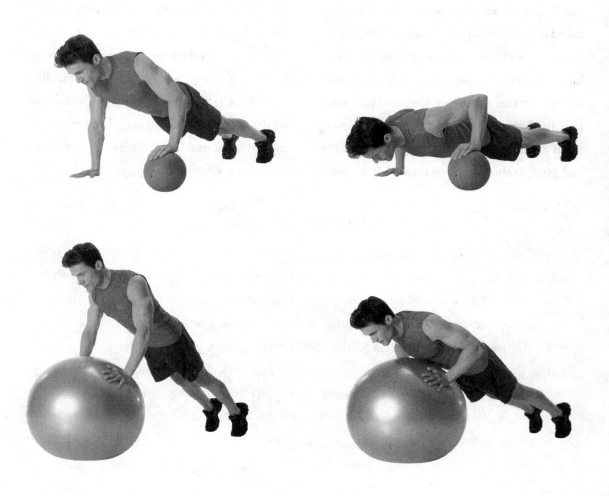

BOSU Pushup and Foam-Roll Pushup

Pushups can also be done on a BOSU trainer or foam roll. Start with the BOSU ball turned over, ball side down, and hold the plastic with each hand. Perform pushups in a slow, controlled manner without locking your elbows out at the top. If this is too difficult, practice in the modified pushup position, on your knees instead of your toes.

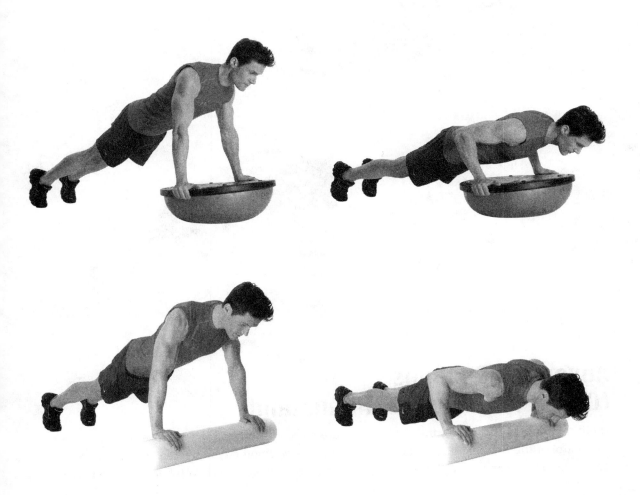

Pushup Plus

Perform a typical pushup with hands either flat on the floor or holding on to dumbbells. In the extended position, arch your upper back to push your body even farther upward.

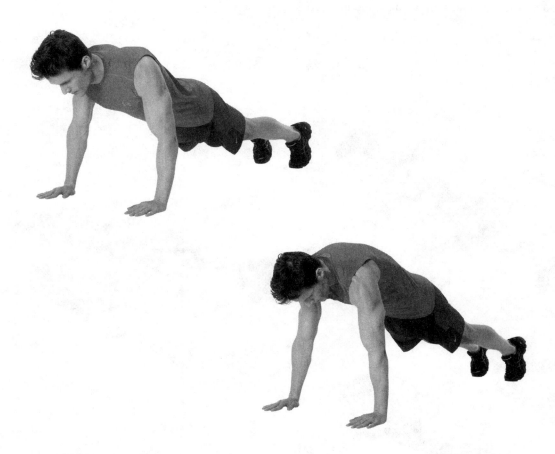

Advanced Pushups (Clap/Plyo, Decline, Handstand)

There are many variations on the pushup that are more challenging and improve neuromuscular control of the trunk and upper body. These include plyometric-type hand claps in the up position, decline pushups with your feet propped up on a bench, and even handstand pushups.

T Pushup
(With and Without Weight)

Perform a typical pushup, but at the top (in the extended position), lift your left hand off the floor and rotate your body so that your left arm is extended with the fingers pointing toward the ceiling. Hold for 2 to 3 seconds, then bring your arm down and complete the pushup. Repeat on the opposite side. To make this more challenging, perform the pushup on a pair of light dumbbells and, once in the extended position, slowly lift the dumbbell up, toward the ceiling, once in the extended position.

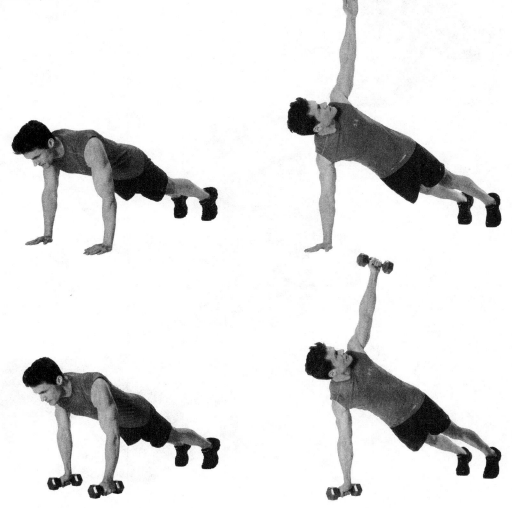

Stepup Pushup and Crossover Step

Start in the up position of a standard pushup adjacent to a step (or a low, stable bench or platform). "Step up" with your left hand and then your right, then down with your right and then your left. You can even try walking across (third photo), especially on a small, stable platform like an aerobic step platform. Work up to 3 sets of 15 reps.

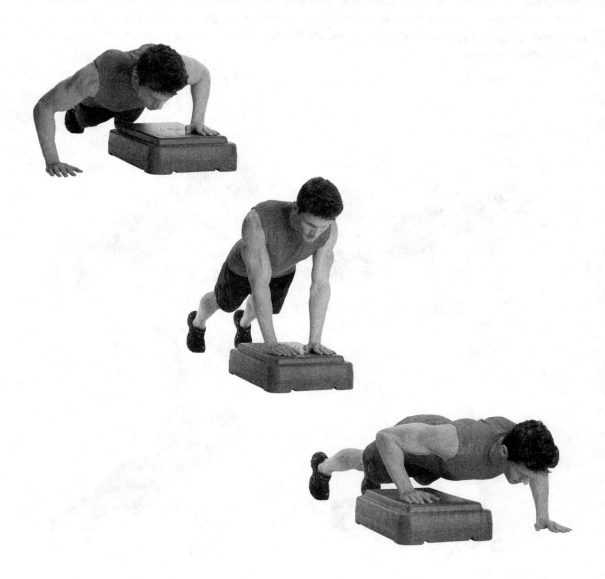

Plank with Dumbbell Row

Start in the standard pushup position with each hand on a dumbbell. Once up in the extended position, slowly bring the left dumbbell up toward your chest, pausing for a second before letting it down. Now lift the right, pause, and let it down. While maintaining the extended position, alternate lifting the dumbbells until you perform 10 to 12 repetitions on each side. If this is too difficult, you can try an incline version (single-arm plank row), starting the pushup with one hand resting on a stable bench (see alternate photo) while the other does a set of 10 to 12 repetitions.

For an alternate version, try this exercise (weight in one hand at a time) while supported on a sturdy bench with the other hand.

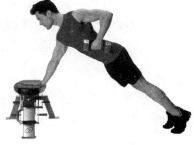

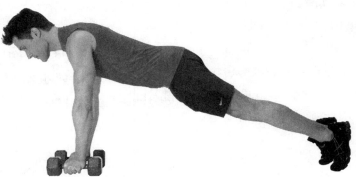

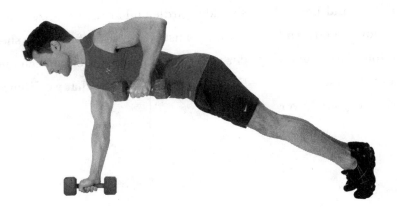

JOINT DISCUSSION

Over the years, I have met many wonderful people through my dear friend Arnold Schwarzenegger. Every year Arnold and his business partner Jim Lorimer (also a good friend and great human being) host the Arnold Classic Weekend and Festival in Columbus, Ohio. I've seen it grow over the past 25 years from a bodybuilding competition to an international multisport event and health expo that is the largest of its kind in the world, with more competitors, in a wide variety of sports, than the Olympics!

One person I look forward to seeing every year is Dr. David Ryan, a chiropractor who works with many world-class athletes, including bodybuilders and strongman competitors. Dr. Dave has an interesting philosophy on shoulder rehabilitation that incorporates rapid-movement endurance training (speedwork) as a higher-level advanced rehabilitation technique. He even helps baseball pitchers recondition their weak or injured shoulders by tossing a ball "backward," which rehabs and works the rear shoulder and scapular area. Learn more at DrDavidRyan.com and read his articles at bodybuilding.com (especially his "Shoulder Fix-It 101").

The next three exercises improve leg strength, dynamic flexibility, and neuromuscular control of your lower body and trunk area, which is the foundation upon which your upper body and shoulders rest. They will prevent injuries to your lower body (especially your knees) as well as your shoulder girdle and arms. I realize you are working muscles pretty far from your shoulder area, but remember the biomechanical links, floor through core, that we discussed earlier.

Single-Leg Squat

Stand upright with your left leg up. Slowly lower your body so your right knee is bent approximately 45 degrees while keeping your back straight. Do 10 to 15 reps, then switch legs and repeat. (If this becomes too easy, you can add resistance by holding dumbbells in both hands, or even try it on an uneven surface such as a BOSU trainer or half foam roll.)

Note: Proper form is critical. Doing this exercise in front of a mirror can help. When first learning to do it properly, try it barefoot so that you can better check for the subtle biomechanical flaws (such as the knee "buckling" inward and/or the foot rolling inward) and correct them. Your shoulder should remain directly over the planted foot. Do not let your shoulder rotate or cave inward; same goes for your thigh. Your foot should not roll inward.

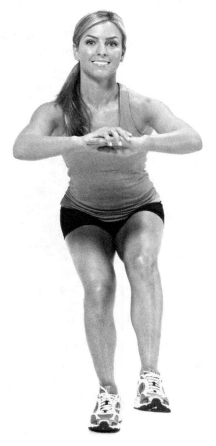

CORRECT FORM

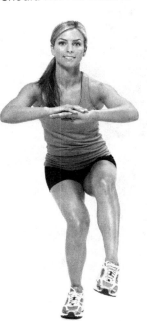

POOR FORM

Tic-Tac-Toe Bunny Hop

Use duct tape or masking tape to make a large tic-tac-toe grid on the floor, big enough so that both feet comfortably fit in each square. Stand on one foot in the center square. Bunny-hop one square at a time forward and backward. Next try side to side, followed by diagonal patterns. Start with 30 seconds on each leg and build up to 60 seconds.

Your right and left leg should perform equally (this is not often the case if there have been lower extremity problems, injury, or surgery). Landings should be soft and controlled and not a "thud." The knee should point straight ahead and be directly over your foot without the tendency to buckle inward or shake.

Advanced version: When the drill on the tic-tac-toe grid becomes too easy, you can advance to hopping over small rubber cones. Include double-leg lateral hops as well as double-leg forward/backward hops. Progress to single-leg hopping over cones. Always be sure that your form is perfect and does not deteriorate with repeated hops before moving to the next level.

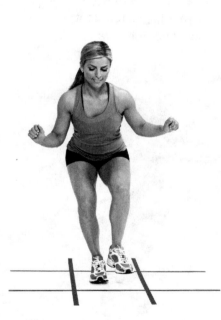
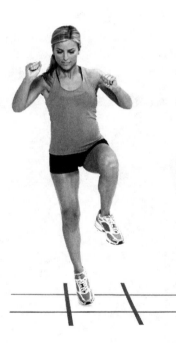
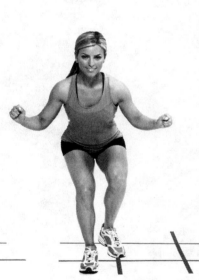

Drop Jump
(see caution at right before trying this)

Stand on a solid box or platform approximately 12 inches high (the bottom one or two steps of a staircase or the stackable steps found in aerobic studios can work as well). Jump off and land on both feet simultaneously (feet pointing forward and parallel—picture a gymnast sticking a landing). As you get better at this test, you can increase the height of the step or platform, and also try jumping higher or onto one leg.

Strive for a soft but solid square landing with your knees bent and directly over your feet. Practice in front of a mirror or have someone videotape you. Those prone to knee injury will land with the knees straight (and/or hyperextended), or they will land flexed, but the knees will buckle inward (toward each other) ever so slightly. Try a few times in a row to see if you fatigue easily or if your form begins to suffer. Also, before trying this on a higher box, platform, or step, you may want to try it on level ground or a small step.

Caution: You should hold off on this if any of the following apply to you:

- Not athletic and not used to jumping
- Don't do sports and don't plan to
- Knee is painful or swollen or has instability issues
- Lower extremity is weak and/or has had recent injury or surgery
- Balance or fall issues

In the above cases, a doctor or physical therapist can assess when the time is right for this important type of training.

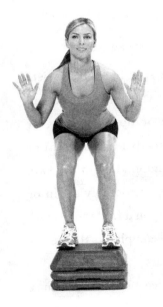
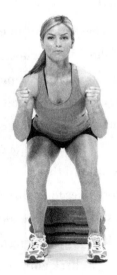
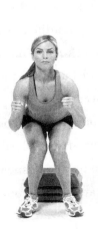
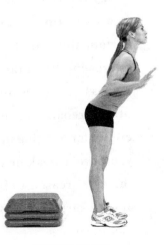

STARTING POSITION   CORRECT LANDING   WRONG LANDING   WRONG LANDING

RECOVERY AND INJURY-SPECIFIC REHAB AND EXERCISE PROGRAMS

While wind sprints can be great training for an athlete, one mad dash can lead to hospitalization—or even death—for someone with a heart problem. Almost everyone seems to accept that distinction, but somehow the same cautionary logic hasn't extended to the musculoskeletal system, including the shoulder region. Some muscle-building and exercise routines, while great for healthy young shoulders, are dangerous for others. There may be nothing wrong with the exercises themselves; they just aren't right for certain shoulder conditions. And there may be other exercises that can resolve or at least improve the problem.

A vital part of the FrameWork program is a collection of exercises modified for certain ailments. This slight adjustment in approach—"the FrameWork Fix"—not only makes the movements safe but also contributes to repair and recovery. So there is no excuse for hanging up your workout duds if you have a weak or injured shoulder. (All the more reason to lace up those sneaks.) Just be sure to incorporate the appropriate modifications.

In every FrameWork book, I've included

an area that helps individuals suffering from a wide variety of conditions to modify their workout routines with a touch of rehabilitation-based exercises, in the hope of improving or even resolving the problem. This is much more of a challenge in the shoulder area, especially with the more complex acute and chronic conditions. Also, regardless of the primary diagnosis, many shoulder ailments wind up with the same functional (or should I say dysfunctional) issues: stiffness and weakness, not to mention pain. So I have organized the rehab and recovery section to help resolve the following common shoulder complaints:

■ The Stiff Shoulder (see page 144)

■ The Weak Shoulder (see page 153)

These issues can be seen in a wide variety of shoulder diagnoses, whether you've had an injury, arthroscopic or open surgery, or arthritis. Almost all roads lead to a stiff or weak shoulder or a combination of the two. And then imbalances predictably set in or worsen. In this section you'll find the Frame-Work fixes for a host of complaints that result in stiff or weak shoulders.

It bears repeating once more that you must always check with your treating physician to find out whether you're ready for these exercises and if they are appropriate for you. Every shoulder, and patient, is different. (Physical therapists and certified athletic trainers are also invaluable in guiding you through the shoulder-recovery maze.)

As mentioned throughout this book, normal scapular strength, mobility, and biomechanics are essential for a healthy shoulder. And if the scapula is sick (there actually is a sick scapula syndrome), chances are the shoulder won't be feeling too well.

Many individuals with lower-back problems will be familiar with the pelvic tilt maneuver. It is one of the cornerstones of lower-back exercise and rehabilitation. The scapular squeeze is the pelvic tilt of the upper back, and learning to do it properly is important in shoulder rehabilitation.

Recovery and Rehabilitation

Recovery exercises are simple, low stress, and yet highly effective for individuals who are in the early recovery phase from an injury, surgery, or anything that has the shoulder down and out, such as tendinitis, arthritis, or some other type of flare-up that keeps the shoulder stiff or weak.

The exercises here will prevent muscle atrophy and stiffness from setting in. They will also help restore balance around your shoulder. This is another reason that we in sports medicine try to keep all of the healthy frame parts active and moving while the injured ones heal. (Remember, also, to try many of these exercises while seated on a stability ball.)

JOINT DISCUSSION
Scapular Squeeze

Stand (or sit) tall and pull your shoulders back like a Marine at attention. While doing this, imagine squeezing your shoulder blades toward each other as if you were trying to hold on to something placed between them. Done properly, this maneuver recruits the scapular stabilizing muscles, including the rhomboids. Practice holding 5 to 7 seconds. Also incorporate upper-back and rear shoulder exercises, especially those in which you "open up" your arms away from your body. Try to incorporate relaxation breathing (page 86) when you practice the scapular squeeze.

Pendulum Exercises

Lean forward, resting your right hand on a secure table or bench. Let your left arm relax and dangle down, letting gravity do the work. Gently shift your weight from side to side so that your arm begins to swing like a pendulum. Do not try to swing the arm; rather, let momentum do the work. Repeat 25 times and then do the same type of movement, forward and back, for 25 reps.

Finish with circular movements, starting small and getting larger as if drawing larger circles on the floor. Do 25 clockwise and 25 counterclockwise. (Another option is to do this same exercise holding a light weight, but remember to keep the arm and shoulder relaxed, as if it were dead, letting gravity do the work.)

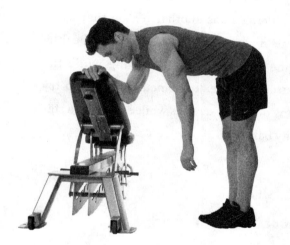 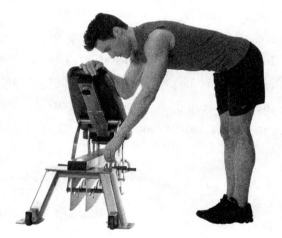

SHOULDER THIS

There is a pulley device that attaches to a door and can be used to help individuals struggling to regain shoulder mobility.

Wall Climb

Stand sideway to a wall, with the stiff shoulder side next to the wall. Place the palm as high on the wall as you can comfortably. Using your fingers, "walk" your hand up the wall. As your hand goes higher, you may need to move your body closer to the wall. Go as high as you can, feeling a stretch, and hold for 5 to 7 seconds. Repeat 3 times. Repeat on opposite side if needed.

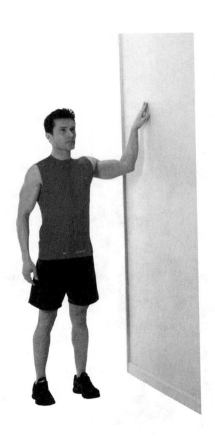
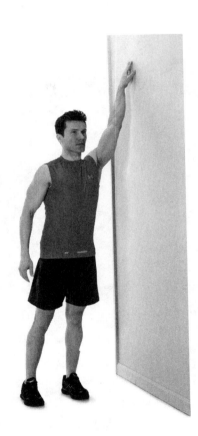

Doorjamb Stretch

Rest your hand, forearm, and elbow on a doorjamb with your elbow at shoulder height. Lean inward, feeling a stretch in the front shoulder. (Picture yourself leading first with the front of the shoulder arching inward.) Keep your palm open and holding on to the doorjamb. This is also a great time for PNF techniques (see page 97). Before going into the stretch, press your arm, elbow, and palm into the doorjamb, tightening your shoulder and pectoral areas; contract the muscles and hold for 10 to 20 seconds. Relax and go immediately into the stretch. Alternate arms.

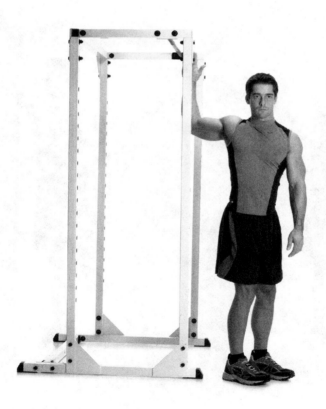

Towel Stretch

This provides a good stretch to each shoulder simultaneously. Hold a small towel behind your head and waist. Pull your raised arm downward (improves external rotation), then use the raised arm to pull the lower one upward (improves internal rotation). Alternate arms.

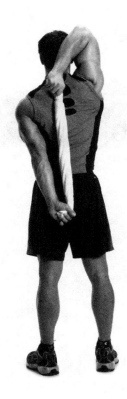

Statue of Liberty

Lie on your back. With your right arm perfectly straight, reach upward as if you were the Statue of Liberty. Hold for 20 to 30 seconds. Use your opposite hand to assist if needed. (If you have a normal, flexible shoulder, you should be able to touch the floor above your head with your wrist and elbow at the same time.) Switch arms and repeat.

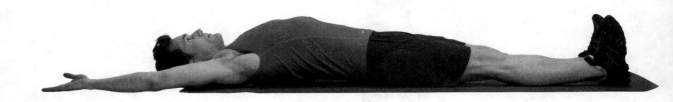

Crossing Guard

Lie on your back. Position your arms out to your sides with your elbows bent at 90 degrees and resting on the floor at the same height as your shoulders, fingers pointing to the ceiling. Gently rotate your arms outward while keeping your elbows on the floor, trying to touch your hands back over your head to the floor. Hold for 10 to 20 seconds. Now slowly rotate in the opposite direction, going inward so that your palms touch the floor. Do 5 repetitions.

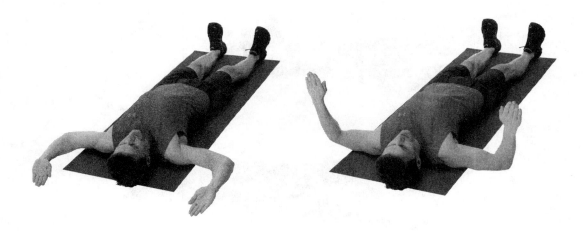

Stick Stretch

Sometimes your stretch needs a little help. This can be done using passive stretching or active assisted techniques in which you use your good arm and a prop to help regain lost mobility in the tight shoulder.

Lie on your back on the floor and hold a stick, light broom, or cane with both hands. Use the stick to assist the stretch. This can be used in different positions (Statue of Liberty or Crossing Guard) to help work out tight areas.

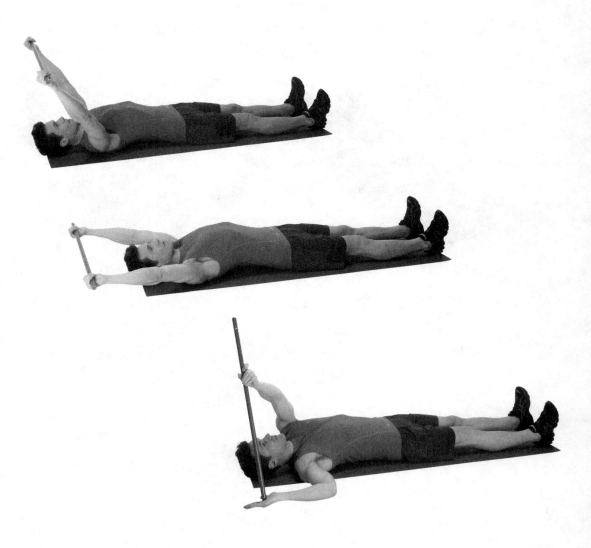

Sleeper Stretch

This is an important stretch for those with a tight posterior (rear) shoulder capsule. Lie on your right side with your right arm against the floor and perpendicular to your body. Keeping your elbow flexed at 90 degrees, use your left arm to gently but steadily push your right forearm/wrist area toward the floor as far as it can go without forcing. Relax, breathe comfortably, and hold for 20 seconds. Ideally, your forearm will be able to rest flat on the floor, but if your shoulder's posteroinferior capsule is tight, it will not go all the way. Incorporate PNF techniques (page 97) to help regain mobility. To enhance the stretch, you can try it with your elbow propped on a pillow or foam roll. Switch sides and repeat with your left arm. If it is more comfortable, you can also rest your head on a pillow.

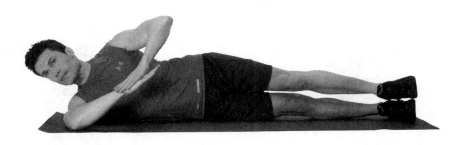

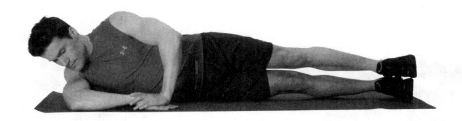

I-Y-T Stretches
(Using Foam Roll, Towel, or Ball)

Lie on the floor with your legs straight. Slowly extend both arms parallel and upward over your head, forming the letter I—like a football referee signaling a touchdown. Hold for 5 to 7 seconds, feeling a stretch in the front of your shoulders. Next, bring your arms outward into a Y position, then a T, feeling the stretch and holding each for an additional 5 to 7 seconds. Breathe comfortably throughout the stretches and repeat 3 times. (This same sequence of exercises can be done on a stability ball or with a foam roll or a rolled towel between your shoulder blades to enhance the stretch.)

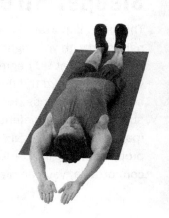

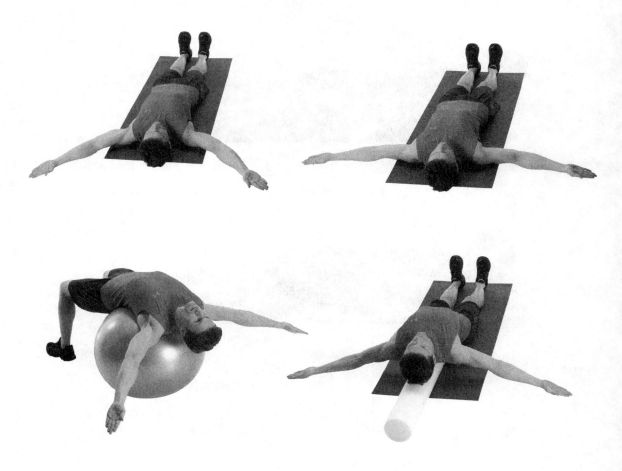

External Rotation (ER) and Internal Rotation (IR)

These exercises (along with the "Empty Can" on page 154) are essential rotator cuff strengthening exercises. Fasten elastic tubing to a doorknob or other stationary object. Lock your right elbow to your side and do not lift it off during these exercises. (To ensure proper form, place a small towel between your elbow and your side the first few times; if the towel drops, you're cheating.) With your elbow flexed to 90 degrees and locked in, slowly rotate your arm outward (ER) fully, pausing in the fully rotated position, then return to the starting position. Do 3 sets of 10 to 12 reps. Change your stance to alter the starting position and use the same arm for inward movement (IR) against resistance.

Alternate: These exercises can also be done using dumbbells while lying on your side on a weight bench or with an adjustable-weight pulley system.

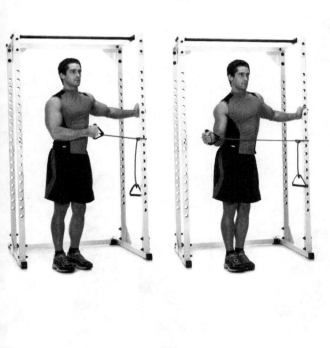

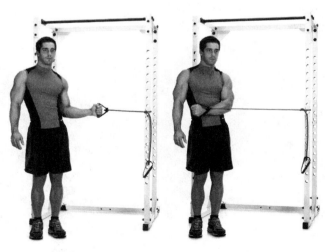

Supraspinatus (SS) "Empty Can"

To isolate and strengthen the important supraspinatus rotator muscle, stand on elastic tubing with your right foot, leaving enough slack to be able to pull the tubing from your waist area to your shoulder. Hold the tubing thumb down (as if you were emptying a can) with your entire right arm forward about 30 degrees. Gently and slowly lift your arm (keeping the thumb pointing down) until your hand comes up almost but not fully to shoulder height. Do 15 reps. Switch sides and repeat.

This exercise can also be done with a very light dumbbell (1 or 2 pounds) or an adjustable-weight pulley system. When the little but very important supraspinatus muscle is isolated, it doesn't take much weight or resistance to strengthen it or strain it—so start light and progress slowly.

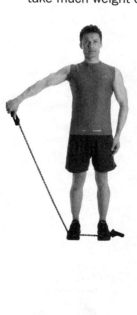
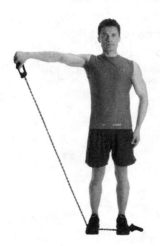

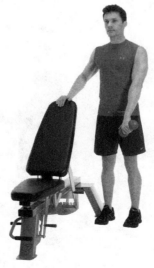
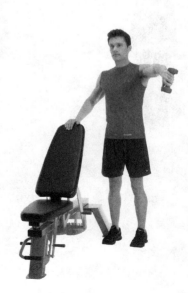

Bow and Arrow

Hold elastic tubing tightly with your left arm extended and your right hand in front of your chest. Keeping your right elbow higher than your right shoulder, pull back on the tubing with your right hand but actually feel the motion lead from your right elbow heading backward. Pull until you are in the fully extended position, as if you were squeezing your shoulder blades together, by pulling both shoulders backward. Your left hand and right elbow should be slightly behind the plane of your shoulders, and you should feel a slight stretch in the chest area. Do 10 to 12 reps on each side.

If there is discomfort in the shoulder, you may need to slightly drop your elbow as you pull back.

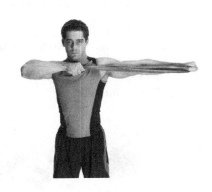

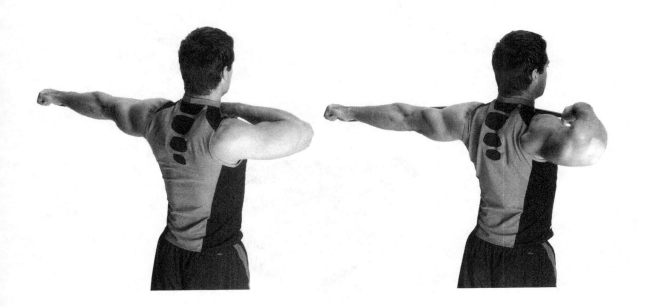

Prone Cuff Side, ER (External Rotation), and Rear Lifts (with Dumbbells)

Using no weight initially (other than the weight of your extended arms), lie facedown on a bench or narrow table. Place a towel or small pillow under your forehead for comfort. Do 3 sets of 10 repetitions of the following six *separate* exercises (Blackburn sequence), using both arms. The lifts should be done in a slow, controlled manner. Don't overextend or force the movements.

1. T with palms down (like a bird flying)

2. T with thumbs up

3. Y with palms down

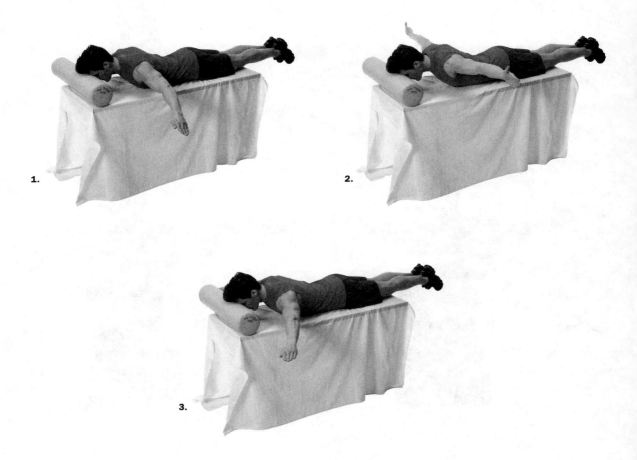

1.

2.

3.

4. Y with thumbs up

5. Elbows bent 90 degrees and thumbs rotating up

6. Arms back and extended along body with thumbs down

These exercises are all relatively short-arc, short-movement patterns that will improve the function of your rear shoulder, posterior cuff, and scapular stabilizers. When they get very easy and are no longer challenging, try adding a 1- to 2-pound weight.

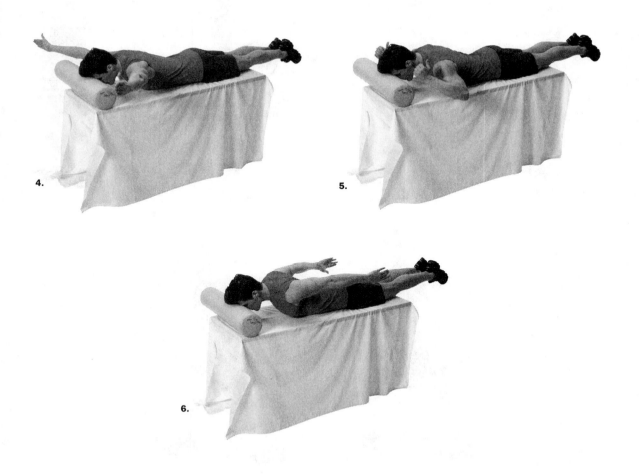

Front, Side, and Rear Lifts (with Weights, Tubing, or Pulley)

Use light dumbbells, elastic tubing (stand on it or attach it to the lower part of a door), or an adjustable-weight pulley system. Perform 3 sets of 10 to 12 repetitions, slowly lifting to the front, side, and rear. The weight or resistance should be very light and comfortable. If you experience any discomfort during the lift, try only a partial movement in your pain-free range—that is, don't lift as high.

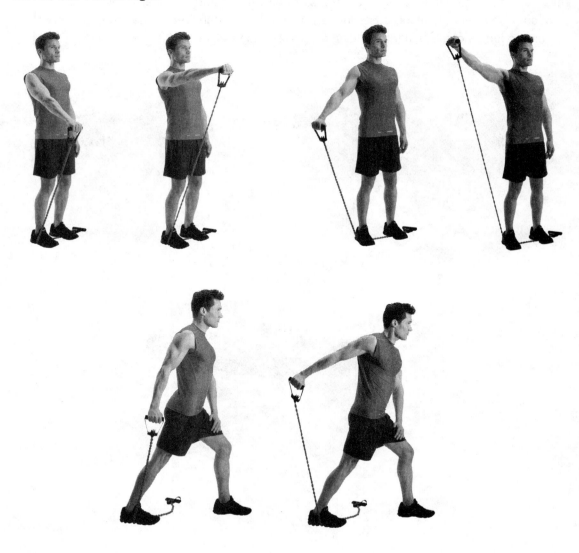

Arm Rotation on Wall

Stand with your back to a wall, hands in the "stick-'em-up" position. Press your hands, arms, and elbows into the wall while tightening your shoulder blades toward each other (scapular squeeze). Hold for 3 to 5 seconds and perform 10 to 12 reps. (To make this more challenging, you can hold elastic tubing in your hands for resistance.)

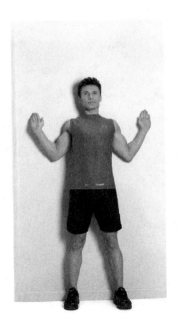 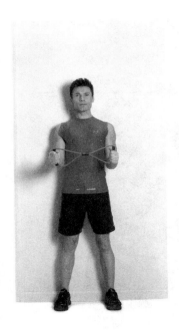 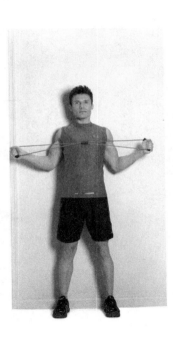

Arm Elevation on Wall

Stand facing a wall with your hands, forearms, and elbows against the wall, with elastic tubing under tension around your hands or wrists. (Your elbows should be slightly higher than your shoulders, forearms parallel, and hands in the "karate chop" position, with palms facing each other.) Slowly slide your arms outward 4 to 6 inches against the resistance of the tubing and hold for 5 to 7 seconds. Return to the starting position. Do 10 repetitions.

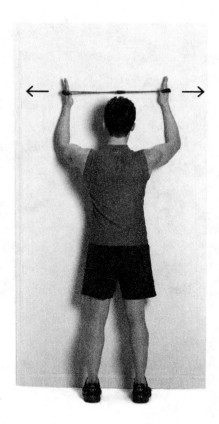

Simple Pushup

A pushup is quite challenging, especially for a painful, stiff, weak, or injured shoulder. It is also a great exercise to strengthen both the shoulder and the scapular stabilizers. Once you are cleared (or able) to perform pushups, you should start with a simple wall pushup. This lessens the weight you must "lift" and thus lessens the forces around the shoulder. When you can comfortably do 20 wall pushups, try to make them more challenging by moving your feet farther from the wall, or do pushups with your hands resting on a stable bench. You can then progress to kneeling pushups, and finally to full pushups. If all goes well, you will soon be able to progress to the more advanced versions on page 132.

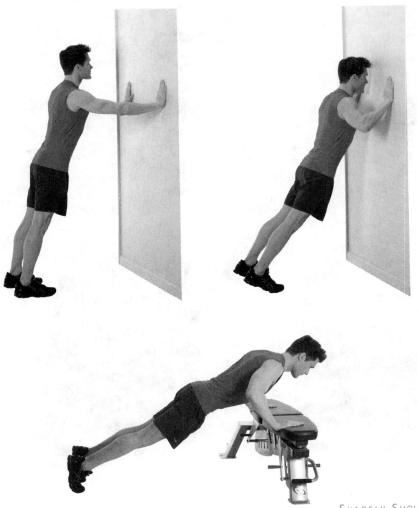

Backhand

Stand with your right hand holding elastic tubing that's fastened to a post or the lower part of a door. With your elbows slightly bent, slowly lift your right arm away from your body toward the ceiling, as if you are hitting a high backhand in tennis. Simultaneously bring your left arm down and back while squeezing your shoulder blades together (scapular squeeze). Hold the extended position for 3 to 5 seconds and do 10 to 12 repetitions. (This exercise can also be performed with a weight-pulley system. Also try it while sitting on a stability ball.)

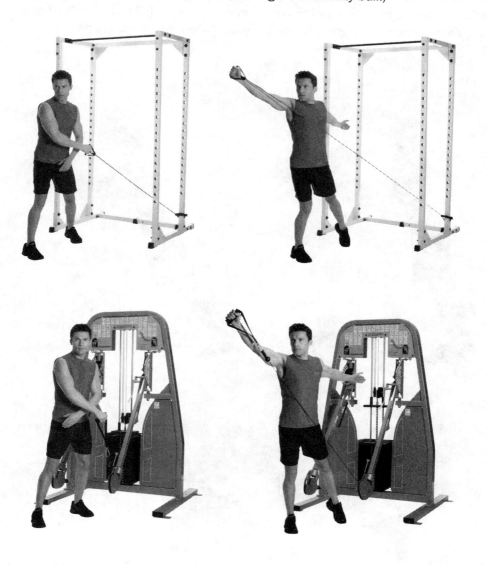

Rear Throw, High

You can add some speedwork as a more advanced rehabilitation technique when your shoulder is feeling better. This should be done with extremely light resistance or a light weight. Stand with your right hand holding elastic tubing fastened to a post (similar to that shown on the opposite page) or the lower part of a door (or a similarly positioned weight-pulley system). Taking 1 to 2 seconds per lift, raise your arm outward and upward at a 45-degree angle toward the ceiling. Do 3 sets of 15 to 20 reps. (To make this more challenging, try it while seated on a stability ball.)

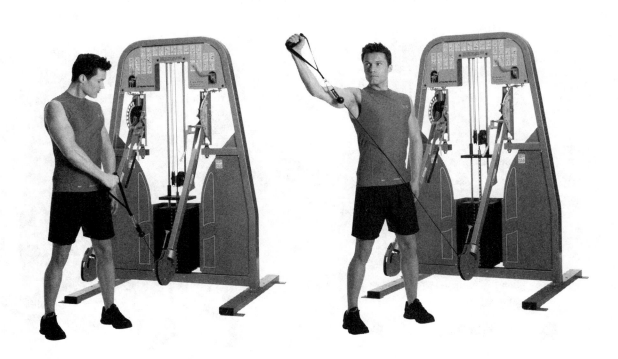

Rear Throw, Low

This speedwork should also be done with extremely light resistance or a light weight. Stand with your right hand holding elastic tubing fastened to a high post (similar to that shown on page 162) or the upper part of a door (or a similarly positioned weight-pulley system, as shown below). Taking 1 to 2 seconds per repetition, lower your arm down and outward at a 45-degree angle toward the floor. Do 3 sets of 15 to 20 reps. (To make this more challenging, try it while seated on a stability ball.)

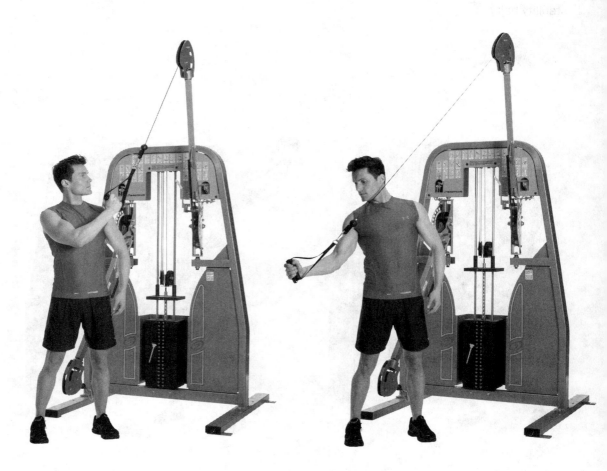

The preceding basic exercises for a stiff and/or weak shoulder will go a long way toward restoring function in your shoulder. They can be done several times per day. As I've said before, if you are having problems doing any exercises, try them in a pool. If you find some that are more effective for you, then stick with those. A little soreness is fine, but you shouldn't be experiencing significant, persistent pain. Once the exercises start to get easy, try to graduate to routines in the other programs in this book.

Injury-Specific Rehab and Exercise Programs

Share my world a bit—the most common ailments and injuries I see day in and day out. They're the ones this book aims to prevent, improve, or even resolve. (For more about these conditions, see the Resources and Sports Medicine section of my Web site, www. DrNick.com, or the patient-education area of the American Academy of Orthopaedic Surgeons [AAOS] Web site, "Your Orthopaedic Connection," at www.orthoinfo.aaos.org.)

JOINT DISCUSSION
The "Unbalanced" Shoulder

As we've discussed, shoulder imbalances come in many varieties and are extremely common. If they haven't already, they will get you in trouble. I see them in sedentary folks as a result of disuse and postural issues, and also in active individuals and athletes, often from faulty fitness-program design and/or repetitive use inherent to their sport or activity. Imbalances can occur front to back, and this is especially prevalent in individuals with a tight, overdeveloped anterior shoulder and a relatively weak posterior shoulder and scapula. Others may have a tight posterior capsule. Anyone with a stiff or weak shoulder (or both) will most likely also have significant imbalances. Restoring balance should be a high priority, and I mention it again because it is one of the basic tenets of the Frame-Work philosophy.

The exercise modifications and additions below that follow a brief review of each injury should be included in your workout and/or rehabilitation. Remember, rehab-type exercises can and should be done daily, even several times a day until normal strength and/or flexibility are regained and you're feeling good. You often need several sets, especially a warmup with lighter weights or resistance for the strength exercises. The approach is very different from training a healthy, problem-free shoulder.

It's even more important to listen to your body, monitoring yourself for any significant discomfort or other changes to suggest you are getting further into trouble rather than out of it. This is especially true as you start to resume more normal workouts, although I recommend always giving your weak links a little added attention. As you expand your routine, especially as it involves the problem area or areas, don't add more than one new exercise per workout. While you're at the gym, you often feel great, only to be sore or even in pain that evening or the following day. When you add more than one exercise, it's hard to know which is the culprit and needs either further modification or exclusion. This is another instance when some detective work is in order. And again, remember: If you're under the care of a physician or other health-care professional, always check with him or her about any changes in your program.

Rotator Cuff Problems

From tendinitis to tears, this thin group of four strap muscles in the shoulder is the number one problem area for people who lift weights. It's also a huge problem for swimmers, even young ones; tennis and volleyball players; and baseball pitchers—for anyone who does repetitive overhead activity. Interestingly, general fitness seems to protect against this, and those who are overweight or have diabetes or high cholesterol are more prone to rotator cuff maladies.

As we discussed in Step 1, the cuff rests between the collarbone and the acromioclavicular (AC) joint above, with the shoulder joint—the ball and socket—below. The peculiar location is why, with overhead use, the cuff gets pinched between this rock and a hard place.

Rotator cuff impingement leads to tendinitis. The cuff gets inflamed and starts to fray like a rope going back and forth over a cliff. It elongates, and then it tears. Also, with normal aging, intrinsic damage can occur within the cuff muscles and tendons, resulting in tendinopathy. The result is a more vulnerable cuff.

Most exertion and fitness routines favor the front of the deltoid and the biceps at the expense of the rear deltoid, the rear part of the rotator cuff, and the scapular stabilizers, creating muscle imbalance—which increases the likelihood of impingement. Creating a balance in your workout to strengthen the rear cuff as well as greater balance in your recreational activities can guard against this scourge of the overhead slam.

The FrameWork Fix: Eliminate overhead lifts, especially the barbell military press, behind-neck barbell press, and even dumbbell military press. Add bow-and-arrow (page 155) and internal and external rotation exercises with elastic tubing (page 153). Modify side raises to unilateral (supported), and limit arc to pain-free range. Do side-raise variations such as supraspinatus (empty can) strengthening (page 154). Add the rear cuff lateral raise (page 156) and sleeper stretch (page 151). Do rotator cuff stretches like the pillar stretch, arm cross stretch, doorjamb stretch, and TriSho stretch that we introduced in the Flexibility section above.

As your shoulder improves, you can gradually begin to introduce other lifts, but remember: You may be prone to develop this again. When resuming overhead lifts, first try the dumbbell military press with very light weights. If symptoms return, cut back to this fix.

Shoulder Instability

As we've discussed before, shoulders can be loose and even unstable. This commonly occurs after an injury in which the shoulder subluxes or dislocates. Sometimes it occurs without injury, because some individuals have joint laxity as a result of their genetics. The far majority of loose shoulders slip out anteriorly, although some have posterior instability and even multidirectional instability. Most individuals know their vulnerable position, where the shoulder feels like it may slip, or their treating physician or therapist can advise them in this regard. This becomes very important in outlining safe exercise routines.

Exercise can be quite helpful in strengthening the supporting muscles around the shoulder, thus lessening the risk of instability episodes. However, certain common exercise-related positions can put the shoulder at risk. The key is to try to strengthen the shoulder to better protect it from slipping out of its socket and to keep it in a safe range of motion. This usually includes working in a limited arc of movement away from the vulnerable positions. Elastic tubing (pages 153, 154, and 158) and scapular-stabilizing exercises (pages 155, 156, 157, 159, and 160) are usually well tolerated.

Even though the shoulder may be loose in one area, there can still be tightness elsewhere. This is often seen in the anterior instability pattern, in which the posterior capsule may be too tight. So stretching is helpful, but the same precautions exist, avoiding the vulnerable positions.

Physical therapists can help you through this somewhat tricky maze. For those who don't respond to exercise and rehabilitation, and for whom instability continues to be a problem, surgery is usually necessary. Postoperatively, you will be guided through many of the exercise routines and precautions noted in this section.

Shoulder Arthritis

As we have said before, the incidence of shoulder arthritis is sharply on the rise, and arthritis is the number one cause of activity limitation in adults in our nation. Unfortunately, we are also seeing it in younger and younger patients. Pain, stiffness, and weakness are all common, and patients often find themselves in a downward spiral and that vicious cycle we mentioned earlier. It is essential to break that cycle, and exercise is one of the keys—but it must be done in a way so as to not overly irritate the shoulder.

Temporary, relatively mild discomfort is to be expected, and if you can work through that, you will improve. No two shoulders are alike when it comes to arthritis, and what works for someone else may not work for you. Also, depending on the location of the arthritis within your shoulder (i.e., glenohumeral joint main socket or AC joint/end of collarbone), some activities and exercises are better tolerated, and some will precipitate a flare-up. So you need to monitor things and be prepared to make some adjustments. (For example, the bench press can aggravate AC joint problems.)

The FrameWork Fix: For glenohumeral joint (the main shoulder socket) arthritis, motion loss (and pain) is the primary problem. Muscle weakness quickly follows. The initial goal is to regain shoulder motion, or at least prevent further loss. Start with a good overall aerobic warmup to get blood flowing through the shoulder area. Next, do pendulum exercises (page 144). Follow this with gentle stretching (pages 144 to 152) that your shoulder tolerates.

The key is to work gently and within your comfort range and not to force anything. If you have access to a pool, performing the motion exercises in a water environment is very comforting to a sore shoulder and enhances your ability to regain motion comfortably, as your arm weighs less and moves more easily while feeling supported.

Perform rotator cuff tubing exercises (pages 153 and 154) and some light dumbbell strengthening within your pain-free shoulder range of motion—that is, what you can comfortably get without forcing.

For AC joint arthritis, most of the usual exercise routines outlined earlier in this chapter can be performed, but there is often difficulty with the bench press and pushup. Try to vary the width of your grip for these exercises and try some of the newer handles available for pushups.

For both glenohumeral and AC arthritis, just as it is important to warm up properly, you should cool down your shoulder area with ice for 15 to 20 minutes after your exercise routine.

Pre– and Post–Shoulder Replacement

Shoulder-replacement surgery (TSA, or total shoulder arthroplasty) has emerged as a relatively new option for individuals suffering from shoulder arthritis, for those with the long-term consequence of a badly torn rotator cuff, or for those with certain fractures around the shoulder. Newer shoulder-replacement designs and techniques have resulted in much better functional results for those undergoing the surgery. The results are not quite on par with knee and hip replacements, but we are rapidly getting there.

With the right pre- and postoperative exercise routines, I believe shoulder-replacement patients can enjoy even more success than those who've had their hips or knees replaced. Unfortunately, many joint-replacement surgeons fail to optimize their patients' functional results by not focusing more on exercise and fitness. I think this is beginning to change, but not fast enough for me.

Many patients with arthritis, especially the elderly, have become very weak and deconditioned because of pain and inactivity, and I don't just mean their shoulders. The weakness involves their entire bodies: musculoskeletal structure, cardiovascular system, metabolism. Many are overweight. Many are in too much pain preoperatively to work on their fitness, but that is where physical therapy, and perhaps a water-based program, can help. The stronger and more fit you are going into the surgery, the quicker and more complete your recovery will be. Certainly, a priority afterward should be not only to regain optimal shoulder function but to improve overall health and fitness.

The FrameWork Fix: After the surgery, shoulder rehabilitation and overall fitness are essential. In the early phases, the main goal is to reduce swelling and pain and to regain mobility, especially lost motion. This is more difficult and takes more effort if the shoulder is stiff, with lost motion, before surgery. Physical therapy can help tremendously, especially in the early postoperative period. Once the shoulder settles down, you can focus on regaining strength and endurance not only in your shoulder and leg but throughout your entire body.

Start with the shoulder range of motion (ROM) exercises (pages 144 and 145). Remember, motion is lotion. When your wound is fully healed, you can try water-based exercise like water walking, ROM in water, and the use of a kickboard.

Regaining strength is critical. Start with gentle isometrics, using your normal arm for resistance while lifting the otherwise stationary, operated-on arm. This can be done at different arm angles and positions. Next, add elastic tubing exercises (pages 153, 154, and 158).

The goal is to progress to all of the recovery-type shoulder exercises. Remember to continue to exercise the other parts of your body that are working fine, so that you can maintain overall health even during your recovery.

Shoulder Arthroscopy

Along with childbirth and hysterectomies, arthroscopic surgery is the most common hospital procedure in America. It's most commonly done for the knee, but the shoulder is catching up quickly.

The FrameWork Fix: Although I would love to give specific routines that apply to everyone who has had a shoulder scope, they are all a little different in terms of what was done and what restrictions are placed on you, especially in the early post-op period. For example, if floating chips or a loose body is removed, you can probably get back to full exercise routines as soon as your shoulder feels good enough, usually within a few weeks. However, if a large tear in the rotator cuff or labrum is stitched and repaired, then your progression must be gradual and is best determined by your surgeon and therapist. Usually you will be starting with the recovery routines that start on page 142, and you will also at some point be dealing with a stiff- or weak-shoulder routine (pages 144 and 153). My best advice is to take this book to every medical appointment you have and see which exercises get the green light at each point in your recovery. Some may be off-limits temporarily, or even permanently, depending on your diagnosis and what exactly was done.

Cartilage Regeneration

We have now entered the era of regenerative (as opposed to reparative) orthopaedic surgery, which means that we can now sometimes actually regenerate damaged tissue or structures, including joint cushions. We have covered this quite extensively in this book (and even more in other FrameWork books): It is very exciting for shoulder surgeons and their patients alike. There are several procedures that can be used to try to regrow injured or damaged shoulder cushions, and the two that are most commonly performed are microfracture surgery and autologous chondrocyte implantation or transplantation (ACI). Both are still relatively new to the shoulder, with a much longer established track record in the knee.

Microfracture surgery, developed by my friend and one of my mentors, Dr. Richard Steadman, in Vail, Colorado, is a relatively simple arthroscopic outpatient procedure that counts on your body's own stem cells to patch the damaged area. However, ACI is a more involved open surgery in which your own cartilage cells are actually implanted after having been grown in the laboratory.

In both types of surgery, the recovery is relatively slow, and a staged progressive rehabilitation program is critical and every bit as important as the surgery itself. Often, patients have more difficulty with the postoperative restrictions and rehabilitation than with the actual surgery. People do not like restrictions placed upon them, especially if they (and their shoulders) are feeling well, but this is one time when your body can deceive you. You might feel well pretty quickly, but the inside of your shoulder is not ready for prime time. It takes tremendous patience; failure to follow your rehab protocol can result in suboptimal results.

More-specific rehabilitation programs for

microfracture can be found at Dr. Steadman's Web site (www.steadman-hawkins.com). Also, information about chondrocyte transplantation can be found at www.carticel.com.

The FrameWork Fix: Start with recovery exercises like simple pendulum exercises, gentle stretching, and strengthening with light elastic tubing. When you get the green light from your surgeon, who will also probably recommend a continuous passive motion (CPM) machine or device to optimize cartilage regrowth, move on to more challenging exercises that are comfortable for you.

Incorporate water-based shoulder exercise for the reasons described in the shoulder arthritis section above. I do not recommend any higher-impact loading for approximately 9 months, because the newly formed joint cushion needs adequate time to mature and become more durable. During the shoulder recovery period, you can continue to strengthen your opposite arm and work on your core and your lower-extremity strength and flexibility. The full cycle of shoulder cushion regrowth and maturation can take up to 2 years, so you must be extremely patient. We're hoping that we can accelerate this process with the new cell therapies on the horizon.

Neck Strains and Degenerative Disease

As I've said before, neck dysfunction is very common in individuals with shoulder problems, as they often go hand-in-hand. Like lower-back pain, neck trouble can be the result of simple repetitive strain from typing on a computer or even just leaning over paperwork. Old sports injuries and auto accidents are also a huge factor in the prevalence of this condition. Football, even in teenagers, takes a heavy toll on the cervical spine. At the gym, too many of us "do in" our necks trying to go for that extra repetition on a shoulder press or a pulldown machine. All it takes is one sudden straining of the neck to create the weak link that then becomes a lifelong problem. And quite often, if the neck is malfunctioning, it takes its toll on the shoulder and vice versa. The two areas are intimately connected, for better and for worse

There is much you can do to avoid this kind of injury. A simple neck-protection approach that's appropriate for most people is lowering one's general stress level. (The same holds true for the back, which is notorious for harboring and abetting stress.) I can't send you off to Rancho Relaxo, but I can "stress" the importance of becoming more aware of how

Neck Isometrics

Interlace your fingers and clasp your hands behind your head and push your head backward, but resist the movement with your hands, tightening your neck extensor (back-of-neck) muscles. Hold for 5 to 7 seconds. Repeat 5 times.

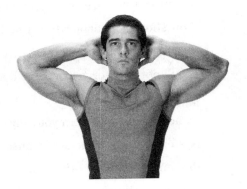

Next, press against your forehead as you lean your head forward. Then press on the left and right sides of your head as you lean to each side.

Isotonic (moving) alternative: Elastic tubing can be used, allowing a small amount of motion—rather than an isometric hold—to be added. This is done by placing the elastic band against your head for resistance. Keep the movement slow and within your pain-free range.

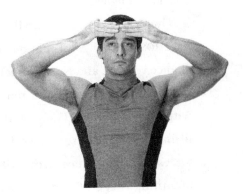

Gym alternative: Seek out four-way neck machines; start with no weight and work in your pain-free range.

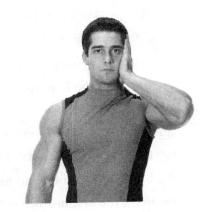

and where you carry tension in your body and the proper posture and alignment to offset it. You should incorporate a few basic mind-body techniques (outlined in the previous step), not only for your neck but also to lower your potential for developing a stress-related condition anywhere in your musculoskeletal system. Massage and other muscle-relaxation techniques, among other options available to you, go a long way.

The FrameWork Fix: Do the Neck Roll on page 102 as a range-of-motion exercise every chance you get, and Neck Isometrics for neck strength. Add upper-body strengthening, but with lower weight and unilateral reps. Modify lifting technique to reduce neck-compression forces. Help to reduce stress with relaxation breathing (page 86) and aerobic workouts. (Walking and elliptical machines are ideal for that.) Swimming can be problematic, so vary your stroke if you are a swimmer. If you are a cyclist, raise the handlebar (extensions are available at most bike shops), and also consider brake extensions so that if you are holding the upper center area of the handlebar, the brakes are within your grip rather than requiring you to lean down to the usual hand-grip/brake area.

SHOULDER THIS

A few final rehab reminders:

- Warm up before exercising.
- Do 3 sets of 10 to 12 reps.
- Never sacrifice good form for amount of weight or resistance.
- Try many of the exercises while seated on a stability ball.
- Ice down afterward.
- Be patient! Gains will come.

If these problems persist, see a spine specialist for proper evaluation and recommendations.

BUILT TO LAST

If you've been lucky enough to avoid a major shoulder injury so far, congratulations. Unfortunately, time itself is causing changes in your body that make at least one injury far more likely to become your companion in the future.

Again, the FrameWork program is all about extending the warranty on your frame. If you have any musculoskeletal ailment, get it checked out sooner rather than later. Often a simple rehabilitation program can get you out of trouble, or keep it from getting worse while you heal.

Better yet, put prevention to work *now*. Monitor your body for signs and symptoms of frame-related ailments. Also, perform the self-test regularly so you can nip things in the bud before they sideline you. The FrameWork program offers plenty of protection from most musculoskeletal problems so that you can count on being more durable for life, with a frame that is solid and a body that's built to last.

"Shouldering" an Active Life

Whether you define *active* as being able to play competitive singles tennis or simply being able to move about and perform your usual daily tasks, you'll be active for life if you commit to a regular workout program. The specifics and level of your physical fitness are unique to you, but *action* is something that applies to every case.

Hurting or not, your frame requires attention if it is to recover from injury and stay healthy. *What* you are able to do to support it isn't as important as doing *something*. The whole idea is to engage in the appropriate targeted exercises—the ones you can tolerate—and progress at your own pace. Remember, this is not a competition.

It sometimes takes a little detective work to determine which exercises are best for your situation and which you should avoid. Use the ones that work best for you more often and refrain from doing those that cause significant discomfort (but don't forget to cautiously and gently try them again later when your shoulder improves). Over time, and with some trial and error, you will probably develop your own optimal routine, as this is not a one-size-fits-all program.

As I have said, if you are having difficulty advancing, try adding only one new exercise per session to see how you tolerate it. Sometimes an exercise feels good while you are doing it, but later that evening or the next day, you're in trouble. If you've added numerous exercises, it is difficult to determine which one or two are the culprits. You might have to stay at a low level of exercise indefinitely, or you might wind up going back and forth between challenge levels, but that's okay. As long as you keep taking steps, however small, your frame will be in far better shape down the road.

Shoulder Scrips

The theme of this book, as in all FrameWork programs, is that you've got to keep moving. With busy lifestyles, that isn't always easy; when discomfort or pain accompanies routine movement of a frame part, inactivity can become standard operating procedure. Complicating matters, some joints, such as the ones in your fingers, are especially prone to getting stiff from lack of use. The shoulder is also in this group.

If you're one of those "tweeners" I often refer to—not a candidate for the scope and not an appropriate candidate for a total joint replacement—staying active can sometimes be quite problematic. Sports and recreation enthusiasts sometimes manage chronic shoulder discomfort or pain by cutting way back on an activity, or by hanging it up for good. If there is no pain associated with routine shoulder movements from then on, they soon grow accustomed to a less active state, much as a couple of extra pounds around the waist results in accepting a larger pants size.

Whatever its cause, inactivity is a prescription for trouble. It is one of those setups we talked about, and it leads to the downward spiral that we discussed in that step.

The information that follows will help those with ongoing shoulder problems or issues, and it wouldn't hurt for everyone to be familiar with what age or circumstance may have in store. It covers the nonsurgical steps you can take, alone or in combination with a professional, that may improve how your shoulder feels or functions on a day-to-day basis no matter what your starting point is.

The one constant that should inform all your efforts to get better is that every step you take should be one that leads to improved function, maximum activity, and more enjoyment of life at every stage. If you can barely move a shoulder, 50 percent of routine function

JOINT DISCUSSION

I have a lot of middle-aged patients who are accustomed to doing heavy-duty workouts and have trouble accepting the fact that their shoulders have changed in multiple ways: Muscle has lost some fiber, soft tissue has lost some elasticity, bones may be weaker, vascularity is diminished, and nerves don't fire as rapidly as they once did. Telling someone to cut back on an activity is always a last resort for me. That being said, I spend a lot of time trying to explain to these patients that they're headed for real trouble if they keep doing what they're doing without focusing on shoring up their shoulders and thinking a little differently about their frames.

Ultimately, we all must make some concessions to age. I didn't really start paying attention to my shoulder until I turned 50, when some stuff I did in the gym all the time, such as overhead presses, had to be modified to avoid discomfort from an aging rotator cuff and some impingement syndrome. I know that tightness in my upper spine and some scapula weakness are ongoing biomechanical issues for me; fortunately, I also know there's a lot I can do to address them. I spend a lot of time telling that to my patients, too.

is an attainable initial goal; if you're at 50 percent, restoring routine function is what you should be shooting for; if you've cut back or eliminated a sport or recreational activity, you can regain most, if not all, of your game.

By all means, you should seek relief from pain with over-the-counter (OTC) or prescription medications, maybe even an injection, but that is only step one in the recovery process—and it has to be a short one, because each of these treatment options has complica-

tions. We doctors know that meds and injections go only so far.

Of import now for all shoulders is that every day we're increasing our knowledge about how important motion and the lotion it delivers are. There are plenty of options in this section that can help you stay on the move. Find the ones that work for you—whatever will give you the ability to move and exercise more. That, my friend, leads to permanent improvement.

END THE VICIOUS CYCLE

You can go only so far with heat and ice and ibuprofen and naproxen, and many recommendations and treatments from doctors have a shelf life as well. It sure is frustrating to be at the mercy of one's shoulder or shoulders, in constant search for improvement. First and foremost in your search is that you won't make much progress if you don't start out with a positive, proactive attitude about finding help. Solutions aren't always immediately visible, and traditional approaches aren't always going to get you where you want to go. I've learned to keep a wide-open mind in terms of treatment alternatives.

Don't Forget First Aid

If the OTC medications you routinely take have lost their effectiveness, switch to other ones or try something new. (Just don't mix NSAIDs. I have many patients who've taken a variety of over-the-counter NSAIDs at the same time. Not only is it dangerous, but no one NSAID can reach maximum effectiveness if there are others on board.) If one is not working for you after a few weeks, it is rea-

JOINT DISCUSSION

The desire for total restoration of shoulder function flies in the face of reality at times. One of those cases involved a lovely 80-year-old female patient who came to me when she shattered her upper arm in a major way.

I was pleased as punch when I got the very complex fracture to heal well enough so that she could comb her hair and do all the other routine things, but every time she came in for a follow-up visit, she complained that she couldn't raise her arm straight up and back. It wasn't because she was a major tennis player or had a job that required such movement; she just wanted to be as good as new. Every time, I'd be thinking, *Well, you've got great functional range and enough mobility to do what you really have to do,* and every time, I'd tell her that unless she was going to be the Statue of Liberty, she was just fine. My staff always got a kick out of how I drove the point home, but that playful comment did sometimes get me a stern look from this energetic senior.

sonable to try a different one, because individual responsiveness to these medications varies; but always check in with your physician first—especially if you're taking them like M&Ms.

One thing that is safe to use while you're taking NSAIDs is Tylenol, and the combination (at the same time, or at different times during the day) can be helpful for many. In fact, to avoid the many potential problems with NSAIDs, I have personally switched to Extra-Strength Tylenol as a mainstay around heavier activities, sports, or workouts, and I suggest the same to my active achy patients. Just be careful not to let the total amount of Tylenol (acetaminophen) exceed 4,000 milligrams per day. That sounds like a lot, but acetaminophen is contained in many other medications, and it all adds up. If there is any question, ask your pharmacist.

I have been impressed with Tylenol's ability to take the edge off my discomfort and allow me to remain active and fit. Tylenol may also be a better choice because NSAIDs have been shown to have some potential negative implications for optimal musculoskeletal healing: They can interfere with bone healing, joint surface regrowth, and tendon repairs. The decision to use an NSAID for sports-related injuries should be driven by the need for anti-inflammatory relief, rather than for pain relief alone, and there should be time limits on use, something best determined by your physician and the nature of your injury.

Also, don't be afraid to experiment a little with ice and heat and with new patches, lotions, and balms, such as Voltaren Gel (diclofenac, a topical NSAID), that appear regularly. There is a new topical treatment (Pennsaid) that combines diclofenac with the old pain-relieving standby DMSO (dimethyl sulfoxide), and it is approved for treatment of osteoarthritis of the shoulder. One diclofenac patch, marketed as the Flector Patch, can be worn all day. Some arthritis patients do pretty well with topical capsaicin (Zostrix cream), a natural pain reliever that, when applied to the skin, reduces and even temporarily depletes levels of Substance P, a pain neurotransmitter. Capsaicin is pepperlike, and it can burn a little and even cause some skin irritation. (A word to the wise: Wash your hands thoroughly after applying it, and never get any in your eyes.) All of these types of agents are worth some trial and error, because they provide relief for many shoulders and other joints. (One exception: As much as I am a fan of the joint supplements glucosamine and chondroitin sulfate, I cannot support their use in topical ointments. As I've said before, they help many individuals, but you need to find a high-quality brand and take it orally, rather than rub it around your shoulder.)

Your Physician and HCP

There are many different types of doctors and health-care professionals (HCPs) who can help your shoulders, from your primary physician and/or chiropractor to your orthopaedic surgeon, rheumatologist, or primary-care sports-medicine specialist. It often takes a "village"—a team approach that includes primary doctors, physical therapists (PTs), occupational therapists, and certified athletic trainers (ATCs). However, if you are not getting better, you must consult an orthopaedic surgeon. They have years of added training and experience with the body's frame and musculoskeletal sys-

JOINT DISCUSSION

I recently gave the keynote speech at a Synvisc national sales meeting. I applaud the firm's efforts and those of other companies to consistently develop new and better products that my orthopaedic colleagues and I can use for musculoskeletal problems, allowing my patients to stay active.

The topic of my presentation was the woeful downward spiral of arthritis that results in a vicious cycle of woe: Pain leads to lack of use, which leads to weakness and stiffness, which leads to less use, which leads to more-serious joint and skeletal dysfunction and, ultimately, overall health deterioration. The function of your frame is directly related to your overall quality of life and your ability to achieve and sustain optimal health. Function and health are intimately connected, so we are always looking for ways to avoid the vicious cycle, or break out of it as quickly as possible. Nietzsche once said that what doesn't kill you makes you stronger. I have come to believe a variation on that theme: What does not make you stronger may indeed kill you.

For the umpteenth time: Motion is lotion. Find someone or something to keep you going, and going strong.

tem. Find one who specializes in the shoulder, because he or she will be up on the latest and best information. Discuss the modalities here that interest you and get some input. Your specialist may think it's time to inject cortisone or a viscosupplement ("lubricant") such as Synvisc. (Synvisc is not yet FDA approved for use in the shoulder, but many orthopaedic surgeons still offer it off label and have been pleased with its effectiveness.) If it's been a couple of months since your last visit, there just might be something new in the way of stim treatments, cell therapies, scaffolds, grafts, and the like that can be offered to you. Maybe there's a new rehab technique your specialist knows about that will do the trick for you. At the very least, he or she should supervise or assess the care provided by other professionals across multiple disciplines with whom you would like to work.

Chronic shoulders demand professional attention, but don't necessarily settle for the first doctor or other specialist you meet. You may connect better with the second or third one, or find someone further outside the box if you're stymied. Sometimes you even need a different kind of second opinion. One thing I've learned from years working with dancers and other high-level professional athletes is that

many sports injuries, especially the nagging, chronic, recurrent overuse variety, are rooted not in a single obvious injury but in technical flaws you bring to the event. I can get most injured dancers better, but often it also takes a consultation with a ballet master skilled in technique to find the subtle biomechanical bad habit that is the root of the dancer's problem.

Ditto for tennis players and their stroke mechanics or pitchers and their throwing motions. Instead of recommending more doctors, more MRIs, or more cortisone shots, I often recommend working with a knowledgeable coach, trainer, or instructor to see why a patient is getting into trouble. There are even centers that specialize in biomechanical analysis of athletes using high-speed computerized video technology. You don't hear a doctor say this often, but in medicine, we don't know everything. Sometimes we have to tap into the knowledge of others.

Improved Lifestyle

Your shoulder problems will get a whole lot better a whole lot faster if you first do everything you can to help matters. If you're battling a shoulder problem without being in the best shape you can be in, you're fighting with one hand tied behind your back. Revisit Step

SHOULDER THIS

Scrips for Chronic Shoulder Pain

- First aid
- See your doctor.
- Check and recheck Step 4.
- Physical therapy
- Acupuncture
- Other shoulder modalities

4 on a regular basis: You simply must eat properly, take appropriate high-quality supplements, de-stress, maintain a healthy weight, stop smoking if it applies, keep alcohol to no more than a glass of red wine per day or three to four cocktails per week in separate sittings, and exercise in whatever way you can.

No surprise that I mention yet again the importance of getting going to keep you going. Time and time again, studies have shown the powerful healing effects of exercise; a recent one touted tai chi and yoga as effective treatments for pain. If you can't handle rigorous programs, keep working at the Recovery and Rehab Program and/or easier levels of exercises in the previous step (with a therapist if necessary). It doesn't matter if you

can do only the first step of the first routine. That's a start to the next one if you keep at it.

Physical Therapy

You might have discomfort when you exercise, and it can be significant at times, but if you work with your doctor and/or therapist, you'll stay on the safe side of the pain-injury line and reap the wonderful benefits exercise provides. Your physical therapist, occupational therapist, or certified athletic trainer can guide you through safe, effective routines and help you get through those painful stumbling blocks we all encounter on the road to recovery. He or she can teach you the important difference between hurt and harm and advance your program when you are ready, documenting your progress along the way.

Unfortunately, in these modern times of health-care reform, too many insurers have created financial disincentives for patients in need of physical therapy. Higher co-pays and limited numbers of therapy visits have resulted in patients not getting the full extent and benefits of therapy that they desperately need. This makes it even more important for patients to learn what they must do on their own to maximize their recovery. Health clubs are experiencing an expanding role in this regard, and I have worked with fitness professionals and personal trainers to help make them more knowledgeable in dealing with clients with a variety of musculoskeletal issues. I have worked with the American Council on Exercise (ACE) to develop advanced education and certification courses ("Your Client's FrameWork") targeting this issue. To my way of thinking, health clubs are a natural extension of health-care delivery and to date have been underutilized in this capacity.

That whole area is getting more and more important with our aging population and aging baby boomers. I am working on a very exciting project using the latest interactive digital technology, things normally seen in high-tech video games, to bring customized smart fitness and rehabilitation programs right into your home. I believe it will revolutionize the way we prescribe (and enjoy) exercise and rehabilitation. The future of medicine is very exciting, especially when I consider the possibilities using technology to inform, educate, treat, and monitor patients. As Yogi Berra once quipped, "The future ain't what it used to be."

Under supervision by those you trust, get active *now*.

Acupuncture

I think it's safe to say that most people steer away from any optional procedure that involves needles. If you're stymied by your shoulder, however, it wouldn't hurt to get a consultation with a respected acupuncturist. Studies with patients who have arthritis have shown significant improvement for those who've undergone this treatment, and the long-term follow-up

JOINT DISCUSSION
Prolotherapy (and Other Things I *Don't* Like)

Prolotherapy involves the injection (usually multiple) of an irritant solution into the soft tissues around major joints. The theory is that scar tissue forms and possibly a "healing" response occurs, resulting in improved stability and less pain for a variety of chronic muscle and joint problems. This treatment modality has become popular in some circles (usually not with orthopaedic surgeons). I do not recommend it. I have not seen any convincing controlled scientific data to warrant this invasive intervention, and I believe that the limited success seen with it can be attributed primarily to the placebo effect. I have seen way too many children with elusive patellar pain syndromes exposed to this treatment.

As with prolotherapy, there are other things being injected into joints with claims they can "regrow" articular cartilage or joint cushions. There are ads (especially in airplane magazines) showing pre- and postinjection x-rays with joint space and cushioning improved after injection therapy. Please don't be fooled by this. These treatments are costly and not typically covered by insurance. Although there is some promising research in this very area, we do not yet have a substance that, when injected, will re-form or regrow your joint cushion. If it looks too good to be true (and if they're asking for cash up front), it probably is.

Power-type bands are seen more and more, and they are worn by pro athletes as wrist bands and necklaces to enhance healing and improve performance. A recent study by the American Council on Exercise confirmed what we all really know deep down in our rational minds—they do not work. That hasn't stopped the big lines from forming at a "band" exhibit at fitness expos like the one I recently attended, where I observed the throng that made a purchase. Along these lines, simple magnets placed around any joint, including your shoulder, have never been shown to do any more than provide a placebo effect. They are still very useful, however, for keeping things on your refrigerator.

has shown that treated patients continue to improve. If nothing else is working for you, this approach might be worth a look, especially if there is an element of neck dysfunction contributing to the shoulder pain.

Other Shoulder Modalities

There are more and more modalities that can help reduce shoulder pain and ultimately improve function. Ultrasound and electrical stimulation can be used for a variety of shoulder conditions, and corticosteroid creams or other pain-reducing gels can be used in conjunction with these therapies. Phonophoresis and iontophoresis techniques can help drive those molecules to deeper tissues to reduce pain and inflammation—as well as enhance healing—at deeper tissue levels.

Muscle Stimulation

This not only enhances recovery, it prevents muscle loss and atrophy around injuries, which is why it's been used to treat a variety of sports injuries. It's the perfect way for those who are in too much pain or too weak to exercise to start rebuilding strength after injury, surgery, or immobilization.

H-Wave (Electronic Waveform Lab) is a terrific electrical stimulation device with a unique waveform. It not only reduces the pain of acute and chronic injuries but is terrific for nerve-related pain. (It is theorized that it enhances healing through changes in microcirculation and nitric oxide concentration at the tissue level.) With acute injuries, it can reduce swelling and inflammation, which results in pain reduction and quicker recovery.

H-Wave technology has also been shown to expedite muscle recovery after vigorous workouts and has led to the development of the Marc Pro device by Electronic Waveform Lab. Marc Pro is available as a home unit and is used by high-level endurance athletes as a natural recovery modality. In the shoulder area it is ideal for swimmers, tennis players, baseball pitchers, and competitive weight lifters. In addition, devices such as the InterX neurostimulator (from Neuro Resource Group) provide a unique targeted interactive neural stimulation that I believe works on acupuncture-type principles. This simple handheld device, seen in more and more training rooms and game-day sidelines, helps manage both acute and chronic pain.

Shock-Wave Therapy and Ablation

Chronic shoulder pain can be caused by tendinitis or tendinopathy (more chronically damaged tendon), and any chronically inflamed tendon is fair game for this "shocking" approach. Extra corporeal shock wave therapy (ECSWT) uses a spark plug to generate shock waves that disrupt scar tissue, similar to lithotripsy, which is used to break up and treat kidney stones noninvasively. By causing microscopic damage to that tissue, new blood-vessel formation is induced in the injured areas, facilitating the healing process. Research results have been mixed with this intervention, so I don't enthusiastically recommend it.

Another new intervention for chronic pain uses radio waves (coblation microtenotomy) to promote the growth of blood vessels in and around damaged tendons. This minimally invasive surgical procedure uses the Topaz device (a small, handheld wand) to repair areas of tendon damage and avoid larger surgical procedures. These technologies are now also being applied for knee complaints and other common ailments, including tennis or golfer's elbow and heel pain.

ACTIVE FOR LIFE

Even if you have been around the block with several specialists and haven't been helped much, keep going back: News breaks all the time, and something just published or new to the market might be the trick you need. (The

stuff that is on the horizon is in the Afterword following this step.) Sometimes it's just a simple thing that can make a world of difference. I can't tell you how many times patients have brought me x-rays that pass with flying colors after a surgical procedure and told me their mobility was okay but that something just didn't feel quite right. More regularly than I prefer, a specific exercise or a specific program was the key missing ingredient.

Remember: *Active* is what it is all about, even if it's only at a recovery level. Everything should be in play so that you can play more. If you have the right physical therapy or rehab program that fortifies your shoulder, you will move better. If you get an occasional cortisone injection, you'll reduce inflammation so you can move better and regain lost strength. H-Wave, acupuncture, stim—they all help to one degree or another in getting you on the go. When you move your shoulders better, you'll be more active—and you'll have a better chance to stay that way for life.

AFTERWORD

If a doctor is doing his or her job the right way, keeping up with the latest advances is much more than a sometime thing. My world is always evolving. When I'm between cases in the surgery suite (a huge chunk of my life), I'm thinking about a paper I just read or how the procedure I'm doing might be improved.

I'm certain the focus in the years ahead will be on enhancing and accelerating the healing process. The future won't be about just *reparative* medicine—it'll be about *regenerative* medicine, too. It won't be a matter of patching an injury or fixing it up the best we can, it'll be how you get back to the stuff you had originally, like the 80-year-old woman in the last step wants, along with the huge majority of patients who visit my office day in and day out.

I can hardly wait to use the advances discussed below, which are in the foreseeable future for our trusty old hinges. And, truth be told, if you are doing your frame work the right way, you'll keep an eye out for them, too.

THE CUTTING EDGE

There's a whole lot of fun stuff going on using the latest techno toys in the OR. At the top of the list is the minimally invasive surgery (MIS) that I've mentioned before. We surgeons are always looking to make incisions smaller so that pain is minimized and the recovery is faster. We biomechanical aficionados know that means that getting back to being active will be faster, too.

Major progress in procedures and equipment, and in the development of artificial parts, seems to occur almost daily in one place or another. Image resolution and surgical instruments get better all the time. Some surgeons are using computerized navigation for both preoperative and intraoperative planning. Robots and remote procedures (with the surgeon controlling the operation from the city where he or she practices) are getting closer every day. Computer navigation is being used in many ORs to allow for more precise joint replacement and ligament reconstruction placement. I must tell you, it's like being a kid in a candy store for someone who knows about primitive procedures!

Stem Cells and BMPs

The broadest front in the movement toward regenerative medicine is stem cell research. Stem cells are structures that have not yet differentiated into skin cells, muscle cells, soft-tissue cells, or other types of cells. This means that they still have the *potential* to become almost anything. By manipulating stem cells in the right way, biomedical researchers can use them as a sort of universal building material, cultivating just about any tissue or spare part needed.

At a company called Osiris Therapeutics in Baltimore, scientists extracted stem cells from goat bone marrow and allowed them to multiply in a glass dish. Then they injected 10 million of these cells into the arthritic knees of goats, and the tissues that had worn away began to grow back. The new cells also slowed the rate of joint erosion, meaning stem therapy holds the promise of prevention as well as repair. This would be true disease modification, rather than our current approach of treating only symptoms.

The same principle applies to the therapeutic use of a naturally occurring substance called bone morphogenic proteins (BMPs), which are produced on various occasions throughout our lives. They "turn on" for the first time before birth, when they spur growth in the fetus. They turn on whenever we are in a growth stage or break a bone. Most tissues heal with a scar that is different from what was there before; however, the healing tissue in bone, largely because of the action of BMPs, is identical to what it replaces. Ideally, we want other tissue to have this same capacity to replicate itself perfectly in the healing process, rather than form scar tissue only.

Scientists have now developed a genetically engineered form of BMP that's been approved by the US Food and Drug Administration. These proteins induce bone formation and enhance fracture repair, and can be used as an alternative for bone grafts in healing difficult fractures and in spinal fusion surgery. This means you don't have to "borrow" bone from somewhere else in your body, because a BMP basically comes in a jar off the shelf. We know there are a few BMPs that have the potential to form articular cartilage and thus re-form damaged joint cushions. We hope that someday soon we'll have the same for ligaments and tendons. Investigators are working diligently to make BMPs available clinically in the office and the OR. The impact is going to be tremendous, with wide applicability in the treatment of a variety of frame issues.

Other Cell Technologies

A platelet-rich plasma (PRP) injection was referenced in Step 2, and it and similar technologies that "juice up" recovery from rotator cuff surgeries, knee ACL reconstructions, and other surgeries are being perfected. *Accelerated healing* is the term, and the goal is to have grafts incorporate in tunnels faster and become stronger quicker. Ditto for patching defects in the rotator cuff. It's been done in a lab setting with animals and is just hitting ORs around the country, but more research is needed to understand optimal use to enhance these and other surgical procedures.

We're also making strides with those rebuilding "scaffolds" we introduced in Step 2 that are used to patch soft tissue. To repair or reinforce a badly torn and degenerated rotator cuff, scaffolds consisting of pig tissue have been implanted with promising results. New scaffold formulations are being concocted in "mad scientist" labs from various bio materials, and autografts (your own tissue) are also being perfected so we don't have to use cadaver tissue.

As for articular cartilage, the autologous chondrocyte implantation (ACI) procedure that we introduced in the knee book has been taken to the next level by impregnating the cultured chondrocytes (cartilage cells) into a bioabsorbable collagen scaffold (called Matrix-Induced Autologous Chondrocyte Implantation, or MACI) or into a patch that can be implanted into a damaged joint through those smaller incisions or even via arthroscopic techniques. (Unfortunately, MACI is not yet FDA approved in the USA.) There are also techniques that attempt to grow a better line of specialized articular cartilage cells with more of the normal joint-surface type II collagen, rather than the type I collagen that sometimes forms and is less durable. These advances we've seen for the knee are also now being used to repave the entire road in any joint, including the shoulder, ankle, and elbow. That is what will be needed to fix truly arthritic, diffusely worn joints, rather than the focal areas of damage that we now regularly tackle surgically. (You can learn more about ACI by visiting www.carticel.com.)

As a "cutting-edge" knee surgeon, I have been very disappointed by our FDA in this very area. They have made it close to impossible for biotechnology companies to bring many of these scaffold technologies, which are widely available now in Europe and other countries, to our patients in the USA. I hope that changes soon, as many patients could benefit from these advancements. Regrettably, the ACI procedure here is still a pretty big open surgery.

Some knee surgeons, myself included, have used a version of the patch that is now available in the United States to make the procedure a little easier on the patient. We use a porcine-based Bio-Gide scaffold (Osteohealth) to patch the defect in the knee, rather than making a separate incision to obtain the patient's own periosteum (paper-thin tissue covering bone) to cover the defect in the knee joint (like a blowout patch on a tire). This patch has not yet been approved by the FDA for use in the knee, but it is FDA approved for other surgical purposes, so it is available for use off label in the USA, and I believe it would be useful for cartilage-regeneration surgeries in the shoulder as well. Bio-Gide has certainly been helpful for those patients who are willing to let us use it in their knees. Unfortunately, the FDA has not allowed the cells to be grown directly on the scaffold, as is done in Europe. I'm hoping that will soon be the case here.

Designer "Genes" and "Gels"

An early report from the University of Pittsburgh suggests that recovery from sports-related injuries involving slow-healing tissues can be significantly sped up with gene therapy that enhances growth factors. A true visionary in this area at Pitt is my friend Dr. Freddie Fu. Someday in the not-too-distant future, treatments for injured tendons, cartilage, or ligaments will be an injection instead of a surgical repair. Your own tissue will be regenerated—like a salamander regrowing its tail.

A bioengineering researcher at the University of Colorado is working on a method whereby damaged areas of articular cartilage can be fixed as a simple matter, almost like spackling a crack or divot in your wall before painting. This technique, not yet ready for humans, is called hydrogel, a liquid plastic mixed with TGF-beta (a protein that makes cartilage grow). The combination is injected into the damaged area, after which a tiny fiber-optic light is shone on the material to convert it into a gelatin-like soft solid. In the weeks that follow, the TGF-beta triggers the growth of new articular cartilage, and the plastic part slowly decomposes, leaving behind a new joint surface. The hope is that these hydrogels will be available for human use soon, because they can be mixed with a variety of growth factors to repair and regenerate other body parts.

Other researchers at Northwestern University are employing nanotechnology for cartilage regeneration. They use synthetic bioactive biomaterials, gels, and growth factors (transforming growth factor beta-1) to promote cartilage regrowth.

The logical extension of regenerative medicine is the actual genetic reprogramming of cells. More and more evidence is being uncovered that shows aging is a programmed biological function and not just the inevitable result of simple wear and tear. Although some dedicated people make strides every day, I suspect it will be a while before we can influence the code for breakdown on a microcellular level. In the meantime, the FrameWork program will keep the wear-and-tear part of the equation to a minimum.

PARTS DEPARTMENT

One of the main goals of FrameWork is to prevent the need for total joint replacement. However, there are times, despite all the best efforts and intentions, that a new shoulder is your only option to stop the pain and to keep you going. If you will recall, the good news is that shoulder replacement enjoys a success rate that is approaching that of the knee and hip, so you can expect to see a lot more of these procedures, with advances unique to the shoulder joint—such as further development of the reverse replacement and other innovative designs.

Excitement aside, joint replacement is a huge business, and, as with any big business, companies invest a great deal in advertising their wares—and more and more, these days that's DTC (direct to consumer). Patients need to be cautious when lured into practices marketing the newest gadget, especially when it comes to joint replacement. Far more important than model or type is the surgeon who is putting it in. Do your homework and find one with an excellent reputation who specializes in shoulders and shoulder-replacement procedures, and does a minimum of 10 to 20 per year of the latter if that's where you are headed. Also look for hospitals that have joint-replacement-specialized areas that include nursing as well as preoperative education programs.

One gripe I have with many surgeons is a

missing exercise and fitness prescription after patients are up and going with their new or improved frame parts. I firmly believe that the essential missing ingredient is an exercise and fitness component such as FrameWork. There's plenty of top-notch biomechanical advice for the taking—and it is getting easier and easier to find and use to your advantage. Certified therapists and trainers are in just about every burg, and as I mentioned in Step 6, there will soon be programs that can be used in the home with the interactive technol-

JOINT DISCUSSION

When I was a resident at the University of Pennsylvania, I had the good fortune of working with a terrific guy, Marvin Steinberg, a hip-replacement guru. Marvin is stone-cold serious and a great teacher whom I admire to this very day. I can't tell you how pleased I am when we run into each other and he tells me he follows what I'm doing, has all my books, and still catches me on PBS. He and Dr. Brighton, who was chairman of my department back then, are like gods to me, and when they make a fuss about my work, it is very special for me. To say the least, I was proud to accept Marvin's recent invitation to speak at a meeting of emeriti and other retired faculty members at the University of Pennsylvania, where I remain involved on the teaching faculty.

I like to think of myself as a somewhat creative person, and reconnecting with a much-admired professor reminded me of a spitballing interaction I had with him long ago. Marvin was among the orthopaedists who pioneered the total hip replacement, and I was more than intrigued that day as he explained the ins and outs of the design and modification of artificial parts. At that time, all efforts were being devoted to duplicating the original socket-and-ball anatomy of the joint. "You're replacing the original socket and the ball," I said to my mentor. "But you're starting fresh—why couldn't you reverse the procedure: Put the socket where the ball is and vice versa?"

The good doctor looked at me as though I was completely out of my mind. "Why on earth would you want to do that?" he asked.

ogy available in a Wii or an Xbox. Count on it.

Studies have shown that patients and surgeons are not always aligned when it comes to expectations, outcomes, and results after joint-replacement surgery, and that bothers me, too. Not only do expectations fuel outcomes, but I believe patients will never have the best possible result from surgery if they remain unfit—in body or mind. Stress and anxiety take their toll on healing and recovery, resulting in suboptimal response to a wide variety of musculoskeletal interventions,

"Just because it came that way doesn't mean you can't improve on the design," I riposted. Marvin got a good laugh out of that, and that was the end of that discussion.

I don't even begin to take credit for the reverse shoulder prosthesis that's now in vogue, but somebody who was trying to improve the design of the initial shoulder prostheses that weren't getting such great results had to have asked the same question at some point.

There was a lot of gray hair (mine included) in the lecture hall on the day I gave my presentation. Marvin may not remember our long-ago interaction, and, again, I'm not taking credit—I never talked to a shoulder specialist about this—but I brought it up then as an example of how thinking outside the box doesn't mean you're out of your mind. It means you're in your creative mind, as doctors who are on the cutting edge always are. In fact, Dr. Brighton constantly challenged us during our year of orthopaedic basic science research at Penn to "have at least one original thought." He definitely helped me open the part of my creative mind that tries to see things differently. The august group of scientists in attendance loved being reminded of Dr. Steinberg's admonition as I related our days-of-yore exchange involving my "reverse-hip" idea. What's more, they thought I was really onto something with my theme of extending the frame's warranty.

I hope you think so, too, and that you'll love the idea so much that you'll apply it—actively—every day.

especially surgery. If you have to go under the knife, make sure you cover all these bases with your surgeon and that you are both on the same page.

A properly designed exercise program— *FrameWork for the Shoulder*—is the answer. Push your surgeon to work with you in this regard. You may be opening his or her mind in a way that will help future patients.

YOUR PART IN THE FUTURE

Gadgets and gizmos are always improving the procedures we doctors do, and the focus on regenerative medicine that is in its infancy will make a lot of them unnecessary someday. But no matter how good things get in the OR, they will still be second best to the original equipment—your frame—that you were born with. Your health care starts with you, and the bigger the role you play in the process, especially in the area of prevention, the healthier you will be.

I'll say it one more time (until next time): Your body was designed to *move*. Thomas Cureton, an exercise physiologist, wisely noted that "the human body is the only machine that breaks down when not used." He's absolutely right about that. With remarkable advances just around the corner, there's never been greater incentive to hang on to what you have by using proper exercise, nutrition, and some simple lifestyle changes—a FrameWork for the best of health . . . and for a long, active life.

ADDITIONAL RESOURCES

WEB SITES

www.aaos.org (American Academy of Orthopaedic Surgeons, or AAOS)

www.orthoinfo.org (Your Orthopaedic Connection: the AAOS consumer site)

www.ases-assn.org (American Shoulder and Elbow Surgeons)

www.sportsmed.org (American Orthopaedic Society for Sports Medicine, or AOSSM)

www.asset-usa.org (American Society of Shoulder and Elbow Therapists, or ASSET)

www.carticel.com (Genzyme Corporation)

www.DrNick.com (Dr. Nicholas DiNubile)

www.FrameworkInteractive.tv (interactive technology and programs for fitness, wellness, and rehabilitation)

www.DrWeil.com (Dr. Andrew Weil, alternative medicine)

www.acatoday.org (American Chiropractic Association)

www.apta.org (American Physical Therapy Association)

www.nata.org (National Athletic Trainers' Association)

www.acefitness.org (American Council on Exercise)

www.nih.gov (National Institutes of Health)

www.physsportsmed.com (The Physician and Sportsmedicine)

BOOKS

FrameWork: Your 7-Step Program for Healthy Muscles, Bones and Joints, by Nicholas DiNubile, MD, with William Patrick (Rodale Inc., 2005)

FrameWork for the Lower Back, by Nicholas DiNubile, MD, with Bruce Scali (Rodale Inc., 2010)

FrameWork for the Knee, by Nicholas DiNubile, MD, with Bruce Scali (Rodale Inc., 2010)

Stretching, 20th Anniversary Revised Edition, by Bob Anderson and Jean Anderson (Shelter Publications, 2000)

The 2003 Body Almanac—Your Personal Guide to Bone and Joint Health at Any Age, edited by Glenn B. Pfeffer, MD; Ramon L. Jimenez, MD; John F. Sarwark, MD; and Letha Yurko-Griffin, MD, PhD (American Academy of Orthopaedic Surgeons, 2003)

Healing Yoga for Neck and Shoulder Pain, by Carol Krucoff (New Harbinger Publications, 2010)

Treat Your Own Rotator Cuff, by Jim Johnson, PT (Dog Ear Publishing, 2007)

DVDS

Your Body's FrameWork, as seen originally on PBS (Sante Fe Productions, Inc.)

Your Body's FrameWork Home Work Out (Sante Fe Productions, Inc.)

Your Client's FrameWork (for fitness professionals and personal trainers) (American Council on Exercise; www.acefitness.org)

PRODUCTS

H-Wave.com (neuromuscular stimulation)

MarcPro.com (muscle-recovery, conditioning, and performance device)

NRG-unlimited.com (InterX nerve stimulator)

NutramaxLabs.com (joint supplements)

TheRotator.com (shoulder-stretching and rehab device and information)

ThermoActive.net (cold and hot mobile shoulder-compression therapy device)

SPRI.com (home shoulder-fitness products)

- Interchangeable tubing system including braided tubing
- Interchangeable tubing system attachments (interchangeable handle and/or dual handle strap)
- Stability balls (Xerballs)
- Xergym door attachment
- Xertube
- BOSU Trainer
- Foam rollers

NautilusCommercial.com (Nautilus Freedom Trainer)

MedFitSystems.com

BowFlexSelectTech.com (BowFlex SelectTech Dumbbells with stand)

TotalGymDirect.com (Total Gym)

ACKNOWLEDGMENTS

It would be almost impossible to acknowledge the many individuals who have helped influence and shape my thoughts and philosophy as expressed in *FrameWork for the Shoulder*. Teachers, medical colleagues, patients, and friends—in the gym and on the field—have all had an impact, for which I am grateful.

I would also like to extend my sincere gratitude to the following individuals: Arnold Schwarzenegger for his friendship and inspiration over the years, and also "the gang" at Oak Productions, especially Lynn Marks; David Caruso, my friend and partner in creating innovative health solutions through technology; Lois de la Haba, my agent, who believed in me and this project from the very beginning; Bruce Scali for his talent, professionalism, and collaboration; the top-notch, enthusiastic team at Rodale, including Karen Rinaldi, Gena Smith, Chris Gaugler, Victoria Glerum, Nancy N. Bailey, Mitch Mandel, Troy Schnyder, and Colleen Kobrick; Dave August, Lindsay Messina, Robert Miller, and Joe Kelly, whose images grace the pages of this book; Roger Schwab for his friendship, thought-provoking discussions, and state-of-the-art workouts and facility at Main Line Health and Fitness; Dean Spragia at Nautilus; the Philadelphia 76ers and Pennsylvania Ballet, two first-class organizations I've had the pleasure to work with over the years and from which I have learned firsthand the extraordinary capabilities of the human body and that, given the right circumstances, healing can indeed be accelerated; Frank Nein for his help and support in cyberspace, especially at www.drnick.com and with the Body ReBuilt interactive digital-technology project; the many physicians and health-care professionals who contributed their thoughts, philosophy, and expertise found within the pages of this book, especially the true shoulder gurus who have changed the way we think about this complex frame part; my dedicated staff, Mary Moran and Barb De Jesse; and most important, my loving, supportive family—Marybeth, my wife and creative advisor, and my children, Emily and Dylan, who inspire me every single day.

ABOUT THE AUTHORS

NICHOLAS A. DiNUBILE, MD, an orthopaedic surgeon specializing in sports medicine and best-selling author, has served as orthopaedic consultant to the Philadelphia 76ers and the Pennsylvania Ballet. His advice has been featured on prime-time television and in the *New York Times*, the *Wall Street Journal*, the *Washington Post*, and *Newsweek*. His award-winning television special, *Your Body's FrameWork*, has been aired on PBS nationwide. Learn more about Dr. DiNubile at DrNick.com.

BRUCE SCALI writes across multiple genres and transforms complex subject matter to make it accessible to every reader.

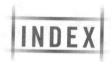

INDEX

Boldface page references indicate photographs. <u>Underscored</u> references indicate boxed text.